CRC
LIBRARY

D0553834

PATHOLOGICAL GAMBLING

PATHOLOGICAL GAMBLING

The Making of a Medical Problem

Brian Castellani

STATE UNIVERSITY OF NEW YORK PRESS

Published by
State University of New York Press, Albany

Printed in the United States of America

For information, address the State University of New York Press, State University Plaza, Albany, NY 12246

Production by Kristin Milavec
Marketing by Michael Campochiaro

Library of Congress Cataloging-in-Publication Data

Castellani, Brian, 1966–
Pathological gambling : the making of a medical problem / Brian Castellani.
p. cm
Includes bibliographical references and index.
ISBN 0-7914-4521-6 (hc : alk. paper). — ISBN 0-7914-4522-4 (pb : alk. paper)
1. Compulsive gambling. I. Title.
RC569.5.G35C37 2000
616.85'841—dc21 99–40431
CIP

10 9 8 7 6 5 4 3 2 1

CONTENTS

Acknowledgments vii

PART I

Introduction *3*

A Note on Strategy: Assemblage and Discursive Negotiations *7*

PART II

1 The Birth of Gambling as a Medical Object of Investigation *19*

2 The Trial of John Torniero *41*

3 Constructing the Gambling Subject: Views from within the Medical Model *49*

4 The Defense's Argument *67*

5 In-patient Treatment *77*

6 Gamblers Anonymous and the Gambling Councils *99*

7 The Prosecution's Argument *107*

8 The Gambling Industry *123*

9 Government *135*

10 Diagnosed Pathological Gamblers *143*

11 The World of Inveterate Gamblers *161*

12 The Family: A Group with No Discursive Voice *177*

13 The Judge's Decision *187*

PART III

14 Epilogue: Addressing the Problems of Pathological Gambling *193*

Notes 205
References 211
Index 219

ACKNOWLEDGMENTS

I would like to acknowledge the following people who've provided me with a tremendous amount of support during the writing of this manuscript. First, there is my wife, Maggie, my world. Thanks Maggie for being one of those people who get it. Second, is my mentor, Dr. Lee Spray, the person who taught me the true meaning of academic freedom and the pursuit of truth. Third, are my family and friends: my mom and dad (Nancy and John), my brothers John and Warren, and my best friends Jay, Ray, Claire and Galen. Fourth, I would like to thank my former boss at the Brecksville Gambling Treatment Program, Loreen Rugle. She challenged me throughout the writing of this book to offer a solution to the problem. Well, Lori, I did. Fifth, I would like to thank the intellectual figures who've influenced how I see the world: Michel Foucault, Anselm Strauss, Richard Rorty and Norman Denzin. Even when not acknowledged, their ideas are everywhere in my writing. Lastly, I'd like to thank all of the gamblers and intellectuals in the field of gambling who let me into their lives to write this book. Grateful acknowledgment is also made to the following for permission to quote their material:

1. "Compulsive Gambler" by Bernie P. and William Bruns. (Copyright line as it appears in the book.) Published by arrangement with Carroll Publishing Group. A Lyle Stuart Book.

2. HarperCollins Publishers (New York, NY), for permission to quote from Bradshaw, Jon 1975. *Fast Company.*

3. "When Luck Runs Out" by Robert Custer, M.D. and Harry Milt. Copyright © 1985 by Robert Custer, M.D. and Harry Milt. Reprinted by permission of Facts On File, Inc.

4. Human Sciences Press Inc., for permission to quote from the following articles: A) A., Paul, Esq. 1988. "Recovery. Reinstatement, Serenity: The Personal Account Of A Compulsive Gambler." *Journal of Gambling Behavior,* 4(4):312–315; B) Blaszczynski, Alex and Neil McConaghy 1989. "The Medical Model Of Pathological Gambling: Current Shortcomings." *Journal of Gambling Behavior,* 5(1):42–52; C) Blume, Sheila 1987. "Compulsive Gambling And The Medical Model." *The Journal of Gambling Behavior,* 3(4): 237–247; D) Bybee, Shannon 1988. "Problem Gambling: One View From The Gambling Industry Side." *Journal of Gambling Behavior,* 4(4):301–308; E) Jarvis, Stephan 1988. "From the View of a Compulsive Gambler/ Recidivist." *Journal of Gambling Behavior,* 4(4):316–319; F) Lesieur, Henry and Richard Rosenthal 1991. "A Review Of The Literature (Prepared For The American Psychiatric Association Task Force On DSM-IV Committee On Disorders Of Impulse Control Not Elsewhere Classified." *Journal of Gambling Studies,* 7 (1): 5–39; G) Ottinger, Paul William 1988. "The Early Warning System That Failed: A Personal Account." *Journal of Gambling Behavior,* 4(4):309–311; H) Rose, I. Nelson 1988. "Compulsive Gambling and the Law: From Sin to Vice to Disease." *Journal of Gambling Behavior,* 4(4): 240–260.

5. And, finally, University of California Press, for permission to quote from Rosecrance, John 1985. "Compulsive Gambling and The Medicalization of Deviance." *Social Problems* 32(3):275–284.

PART I

INTRODUCTION

It was 8:45 in the morning. She was waiting for her first patient. Her fifteen years as a therapist had taught her a lot about addiction. Crack addicts, junkies, alcoholics, speed freaks, she had worked with them all. But not pathological gamblers. This was something new. A fellow colleague had called her the week before saying he wanted to make a referral. His patient, a middle-class, white, female, diagnosed with clinical depression, had asked if someone could see her husband for a couple of sessions. She said he was a pathological gambler. Ruby agreed.

The night before the session, Ruby spent time on the Internet trying to find information. She typed in p-a-t-h-o-l-o-g-i-c-a-l g-a-m-b-l-i-n-g and to her surprise found over five thousand hits. Going through them, she found all kinds of information. "Pathological gambling is one of the most rapidly growing, but ignored, mental health problems in the United States."[1] "Researchers conservatively estimate that 1.5 to 6 percent of the adult population are problem gamblers."[2] "Nine out of ten problem gamblers are men, while 10% are women of all ages and ethnic backgrounds."[3] "Today, research indicates that as many as 7% of teenagers may be addicted to gambling."[4]

The social costs of pathological gambling were profound as well. "Each problem gambler costs government and the private economy $13,200 a year. If you simply increased the incidence of problem gambling in a small state like Iowa . . . by only ½ of 1 percent of the adult population, it would cost private business and government at least 73 million a year."[5] Ninety-one percent of all pathological gamblers in Minnesota are in debt to creditors, with an average lifetime debt of $54,000 dollars.[6] One in five pathological gamblers seeking treatment in Minnesota "had a legal status of either being on parole, probation, or pending legal action as a result of gambling-related legal problems, and 10% admitted to being arrested for a gambling-related offense in the six-months prior to treatment."[7] Pathological gambling also affects the family. There is an increasing need for treatment experts to focus their attention on the impact pathological gambling has on the spouse and family members of pathological gamblers. "Increasing debt, the inability to meet day to day expenses, emotional stress and physical and emotional abuse can lead the families of pathological gamblers to critical stages of desperation."[8]

After reading these web pages, Ruby understood why the wife of her nine o'clock appointment was anxious to get her husband into therapy. He probably caused her a lot of mental and emotional anguish. Their lives were a mess. Her depression a result of it. She was probably doing everything she could to deal with the problem.

Ruby was angry at what she learned—angry both at herself and the problem. How could such an immense social crisis go unnoticed? How could she, an expert for fifteen years in addiction, never notice the problem? Pathological gambling was the silent addiction, claiming the lives of millions of people, and it seemed as if nobody was doing anything about it. Why? While Ruby didn't have the answer, she had an idea. She typed in the words g-a-m-b-l-i-n-g r-e-v-e-n-u-e and found what she was looking for. According to *International Gaming & Wagering Business,* the premier gambling industry journal in 1995, more than $500 billion dollars was wagered legally in the United States. Of this total, roughly 8 percent was kept as net winnings; which amounts to about $40 billion dollars a year. This total, explained one web page, "is more than the combined take for movies, books, recorded music and park and arcade attractions."[9] Why was pathological gambling ignored? Simple, government and business were making too much money. Looking up information just for Minnesota, Ruby found that in 1994 alone "revenues from pull tabs and tipboards were $27.9 million; $2.2 million was collected from the tax on bingo, raffles and paddlewheels, and $27.4 million from the combined receipts tax."[10]

It was now 8:50 am. Ruby sat rocking in her chair reciting over and over again the statistics she had learned from the night before. Suddenly a wave of panic came over her. I've got a patient in less than ten minutes, and I don't even know how to care for him. I have no diagnosis, no treatment plan, no theory, no clinical data. Nothing. What am I going to do? That's when she called me.

I was sleeping when the phone rang. "Brian, it's Ruby. You've got to help me. You've worked with pathological gamblers, right? I mean—yeah—you've had these guys, the statistics said mostly guys . . . You've had them in therapy?" "What are you talking about Ruby?" "I've got a guy coming in here in ten minutes whose wife says he's a pathological gambler and I have no idea what to do with him. What should I do?" "Listen," I said, "for your first session just get the basics like you would for any other addiction." "Okay, but let's get together to talk more." We scheduled an appointment for the following week.

Ruby and I met at a coffee shop in town to talk about pathological gambling. I myself am trained as a therapist. I have my masters in clinical psychology and a doctorate in medical sociology. I worked in addiction treatment and mental health for nine years and spent three years working at the Gambling Treatment Program of the Brecksville Veterans Administration Medical Center in Brecksville, Ohio. During the week following our phone call Ruby read everything she could get her hands on. She came prepared with lots of questions. She wanted to know why most treatment professionals know nothing about pathological gambling and why the federal government has not declared it a major social problem the way it has with alcohol and drugs. She was also concerned about the lack of research in the field of gambling studies. Of all the disciplines within the social sciences, only a handful of researchers—mostly psychologists and psychiatrists—have done research on pathological gambling during the last twenty-five years. And most of it is not that developed. Everyone else has ignored the problem completely. Nothing else has been done. Not even NIDA, the National Institute on Drug Abuse, has really addressed the problem. To date, only the field of addiction treatment has given it the attention it deserves. But this was problematic because they had reduced the entire problem to a medical disorder. As we talked, we realized something had to be done. Someone had to sit down and reconstruct the history of pathological gambling: determine its origins, establish its historical course, figure out when and why it became a medical problem, find out the role government and business played in this process, relate these factors to its diagnosis and treatment, bring in the lives of pathological gamblers and their families, and determine how we can think differently about gambling. Ruby looked at me: "So, you gonna do it?"

Ruby's challenge to me is where it all started. During my three years of work at the Brecksville Gambling Treatment Program, the questions Ruby and I talked about surfaced over and over again. They were important questions. They bugged me as much as they bugged Ruby. I was in a unique position. I knew the gambling literature, had treated pathological gamblers myself, and, as a sociologist, was trained in the various qualitative, discursive and historical methodologies necessary to do the study. I decided to do it. The work before you is the end result of this process. The study you are about to read is an interpretive history of how pathological gambling was made into a medical problem and the social, political, individual, cultural and economic factors that influenced this process.

While this book is the first interpretive history of pathological gambling, it is not meant to be read alone. In 1995 Robert Goodman published an important book titled *The Luck Business: The Devastating Consequences and Broken Promises of America's Gambling Explosion.* It was widely received, including a *New York Times* book review, although very controversial. In *The Luck Business,* Goodman provides a rather exhaustive analysis of the economic and social consequences of legalized gambling. Both the good and the bad. He caused a much needed commotion. However, while Goodman's book examines the social consequences that emerged as a result of legalized gambling, he does not explore how our institutions of social control have dealt with these problems. My study fills this gap. My book is a companion piece to Goodman, and it should be read that way. Goodman reveals the social problems that emerged as a result of legalized gambling, and I show how we have dealt with, or should I say "medicalized" them.

A NOTE ON STRATEGY: ASSEMBLAGE AND DISCURSIVE NEGOTIATIONS

Months went by after my conversation with Ruby. During that time we hadn't talked much. Ruby was sitting at her desk typing on the computer when the phone rang. It was me on the other end. "Hey, how's it going?" she said. "Finish that book yet?" "Yeah, very funny. Listen, have you got a few spare hours to talk. I'm going round-n-round with this book. I really need some help, if you know what I mean." "Sure."

We got together the next day. Drinking her herbal tea, she got right to the point, "What's the problem?" "Well, since I started this study, two issues keep emerging. One has to do with method, the other with theory." Ruby paused, and in a therapeutic voice said, "Tell me about it, I'm listening."

"Well, doc," I said, "it all starts with my method."

"Go on."

"I thought my history would be straightforward, you know. I would study the medical treatment of pathological gambling and outline the historical processes by which it became dominant. But it hasn't turned out that way. I can't locate my study at the level of treatment alone. When I start to think about treatment, I want to write about the field of gambling research; when I think about research, I want to write about the gambling councils; when I write about the councils, I want to think about the gambling industry and so on. It just keeps on going and going. I can't make it stop. It's all so circular, so complex."

"But why? Why are you making things so difficult for yourself?"

"I'm not making things difficult for myself; I'm making things different."

"What do you mean?"

"You see, the medical model isn't the only discourse on gambling, and gamblers and counselors aren't the only forces involved. If my study just focused on the history of these forces, it would fail to explain the larger and smaller histories within which the medicalization of pathological gambling has taken place. It would fail to show, for example, how legalized gambling has influenced medical knowledge, or the ways government has been involved in this process. And it wouldn't even begin to explain the impact pathological gamblers have on their families. In fact, I've never seen a study that compares and contrasts what goes on in the heads of pathological gamblers with the larger historical changes taking place in our mainstream, televisual, capitalistic culture, while at the same time situating these connections within the context of in-patient treatment, only to decenter these inter-actions onto the criminal justice system and other important forces such as business, religion, and the field of health care. And, even if a study did concern itself with these factors, it would still miss out on the influence Gamblers Anonymous and the state gambling councils have on the whole process. And, it wouldn't show the relationship between medical knowledge and the criminal justice system and the heavy influence these interactions have on the diagnosis of pathological gambling."

"But aren't you being just a bit obsessive?"

"Well, it might appear that way. But, I'm not. I'm inducing a different type of complexity, a complexity that doesn't just analyze, in detail, the influence one set of predefined variables have on another. I want to spread myself out laterally to explore in detail the interconnectedness of a larger set of seemingly unending variables. I want to see how far I can go before the whole thing falls apart. Everybody seems to run away from this type of complexity—like it's too messy or lacks control. But it doesn't. It's just as ordered in its analysis of multiple surfaces as any in-depth study of one or three variables."

"But doesn't such a high level of lateral complexity become meaningless at some point? I mean, you can't explain everything."

"But I'm not trying to explain everything! I'm only trying to explain one thing, but in a very different way. I'm thinking laterally rather than vertically. I mean, look around you. In this complex, highly integrated, fragmented, non-linear world we live in today, vertical science offers increasingly limited solutions. How many times have you seen an article that looks at one or two variables, and then goes on—ignorantly—to make some type of policy recommendation? Policy analysts never make such claims. They understand all too well that everything is so much more complex than that. They would never make a recommendation based on the analysis of one or two variables."

"But isn't that the goal of science? Parsimony? Aren't we supposed to peer into the social abyss in order to pull out those one or three variables we find most important to our work?"

"Well yeah, that's what most social scientists do. But, I'm not interested in that. I want to complicate things. I want to focus on inter-action, on the interaction variables have with one another. Not the variables themselves; I'm not interested in that. I'm interested in the in-between."

We sat back for a moment. Both pausing in our thoughts.

"Subvert the vertical bias," said Ruby.

"What?"

"Subvert the vertical bias, that's what you're trying to do. As you say, most methods force us to fixate on one or two lateral levels of analysis while ignoring or controlling the rest. You, however, want to overcome this problem. You approach everything as if it all fits together into one big puzzle. You're opposed to vertical thinking because it conceptualizes social reality as a series of levels, from the micro to the macro—like a cake, one layer on top of the other, fixed in their place, never to change."

"Vertical thinking," I said, "reinforces all of the dualisms that keep each social scientist in her or his appropriate place. Psychologists ignore the sociologists; sociologists ignore the medical researchers; the economists ignore everyone, and the anthropologists are left out in the cold. Everyone is busy doing their own work, blissfully ignoring one another, pretending as if their set of variables were more important than the others. In fact, you can almost define a discipline by the level of analysis it engages in. But I'm talking about more than just cross-disciplinary work."

"How so?" asked Ruby.

"Because, what I'm talking about is a way of thinking. I'm talking about social scientists thinking in terms of lateral complexity (from the inside of the brain to the factors influencing world events) regardless of what level of analysis they choose to study. Social scientists need to be thinking cross-disciplinary in order to continually move up and down the various hierarchical levels of analysis, turning them upside down, sideways and over, inside out. You get it. Like you said, subvert the vertical bias. I'm looking to construct a different methodology, but it's more than a methodology, it's an entire frame of mind, a way of being, a way of thinking."

"It reminds me of the concept of assemblage," said Ruby, "You know it? Assemblage was coined during the 1960s to describe the work being done by contemporary artists such as Robert Rauschenberg. Rauschenberg combined various found and made objects, such as torn scraps of paper, fragments of cloth, forks, ceramics, clippings from newspapers, stones and tires with painting, sculpture, photography and silkscreening to produce works of art that crossed conventional boundaries. Rauschenberg broke the rules, was cross-disciplinary. He disobeyed the laws of painting, sculpture, and the dividing lines between various forms of art, including dance, theater and performance. It seems like you're trying to do the same thing in your work."

"You're right," I said. "I'm trying to bring psychology, economics, history, philosophy and the rest of the social sciences together to create a story about pathological gambling that defies simple disciplinary categorization, boundary, tradition or rule. My goal seems to be to challenge both myself and others to expand the limits of our current vocabulary and range of vision on the issue of pathological gambling to see as much as is possible before things collapse into complete chaos."

"Yeah," said Ruby, "and thinking about your work in terms of Rauschenberg, what I see you doing is glueing pathological gamblers to medical discourses, while nailing treatment structures to state and federal politics. You take attitudes toward gambling and tie them to beliefs about addiction, while integrating the macro processes of capitalism with the micro interactions between pathological gamblers and their families and so on. Structures are torn in half, melted, made into other things. Politics become economics, individuals become organizations, institutions become culture, culture becomes politics, and around again we go. From your perspective the researcher would view the world as non-linear, multi-layered and integrated, fuzzy, grey, polymorphous, non-causally determined, fragmented and disjointed, full of excess and scarcity. The researcher would assume no dualisms, only variations of similarity and difference within the context of a play of forces. And, most importantly, you would ground yourself socio-historically and geographically and wouldn't sell assemblage as a method for all times and all places."

"That's it," I said. "The method I'm proposing is assemblage."

We paused for a moment.

"I was just reading Deleuze's book on Nietzsche," I said, looking down into my bag as I pulled it out. "Listen to this." I read a quote: "'The one is the many, unity is multiplicity.' And indeed, how would multiplicity come forth from unity and how would it continue to come forth from it after an eternity of time if unity was not *actually* affirmed in multiplicity?'"[1]

"Nietzsche's incredible," Ruby responded. I continued to make my point. "In our contemporary society, unity is multiplicity. A study with cohesiveness is a study that embraces multiplicity, not singularity. Vertical method is disjointed and fragmented because it searches for unity through singularity, through foundation or reduction. Assemblage is unified because it embraces multiplicity. Embrace complexity and you find a negotiated unity." "But," I clarified, "not a unity as a singularity, a unity as an endlessly negotiated multiplicity existing in time and space. No dialectic here." "Exactly," Ruby said, "search for unity and cohesion and you find fragmentation. Search for multiplicity and you find unity."

I read another quote to Ruby. "This one," I said, "comes from William Johnston. It's in Magliola's book on Derrida and Eastern philosophy. Johnston says, 'When people meet at the level of personal love achieved through radical non-attachment, they do not merge, nor are they absorbed in one another. . . . There is at once a total unity and a total alterity.'[2] That's what you get when you pursue an investigation via assemblage. You get a study that is at once a total unity and a total alterity, a total difference within unity, a total unity within difference. A multi-singularity." "I like it," responded Ruby.

Thinking we were done, Ruby smiled. I looked into my empty cup of tea. "In case you forgot, I have another problem." "Haven't we solved enough problems for today?" asked Ruby. "But it fits," I said. "I told you I had two problems which were part of the same conceptual cloth." "Tell me what it is," exclaimed Ruby, "but first let me get another cup of tea." "Me too."

After getting our tea, Ruby got right to the point: "Listen, we've got an hour and then I've got to go. What's your theoretical problem?"

"My problem is that I never wanted to just study the construction of the medical model. I've always been interested, instead, in who uses it and why." "You mean you want to know who puts it into practice and for what reasons?" asked Ruby. "Exactly. The medical model of pathological gambling wasn't constructed in a vacuum. It was written to accomplish specific goals in response to a very specific set of discourses and discursive actors already in circulation." "So, you're interested in discourses in inter-action with one another," said Ruby, "as a complex field of assembled relations, one affecting the other, round and round they go!"

"Exactly, no discourse(s), no inter-action. There is no such thing as a single discourse having a single effect; there are only discourses. There is no such thing as action, only interaction. As such, each and every discourse we construct, including the medical model of pathological gambling, exists only as one possibility within a larger field of already existing discourses. There is no one individual discursive will or force, only a play of forces, a play of discursive actors. This is how I interpret my work. I call my interpretive framework *discursive negotiations.*"

"Discursive negotiations?" said Ruby. "Explain."

"Okay. Let me give you an example. Take the interactions between a therapist and a group of pathological gamblers in therapy. Some would argue that the therapist is in a position of domination while the patients are in varying degrees of resistance[3]. In terms of the passage of knowledge, they would say that the therapist dominates the patients by engaging in techniques of normalization, surveillance, and discipline. The patients respond by struggling with the discourses being imposed upon them. But their resistance is in vain, because in the end the story is always the same. The patients succumb to the techniques of domination and become docile bodies which the therapist then controls."

"So?"

"So, . . . it's too limited. It's fails to understand how each patient and therapist exist as the intersection of a competing set of discourses, of which the medical model is only one. It fails to conceptualize individuals as an organized set of discursive practices, where obtainment of authority is won through discursive negotiation. Think about it. To gain a position of authority, the medical model must be negotiated by the therapist in relation to the patients and by the patients themselves. The therapist doesn't just tell the patients what to think or how to act, and patients don't simply listen and obey. From the moment therapy starts, the medical model is colliding with a field of other discourses. It enters into the group slamming into a framework of already existing and competing discursive practices which gamblers and therapists currently exist within to negotiate their worlds. As such, there is no straightforward medical domination taking place. The medical model is neither imposed or applied. It's negotiated. And because it is negotiated, discursive control and power are never complete. Domination is never fully accomplished. Have you ever watched patients use the medical model to manipulate staff or their families? They're pretty damn good at it. They say one thing one day and another the next. They use the medical model to their advantage, even the healthy ones. And this is only the beginning. How about the way in-patient treatment programs change their definitions of medicine to accommodate the economic and organizational challenges of the changing health care system? The more you start to think about the process, the less it appears as if the medical model is a simple top-down form of domination."

"What do you see, then?"

"More of what I see is a system of multiple actors—actors being defined as institutions and professions, as well as individuals and groups. I see a system of multiple actors all engaged in a series of manipulations, all intent on accomplishing their various agendas, using discourses to make certain and various things known to themselves and others. I see people distorting, misrepresenting, exaggerating, and breaking apart discourse in order to come to agreement with others about how best to define, understand and then interact on a given issue."

"It's all a big game of discursive negotiations" said Ruby.

"Exactly."

Ruby thought for a moment, then looked at me. "But what about conflict? I mean, certainly everyone isn't equally involved in the games of negotiation. Doesn't your concept devalue, in a way, the reality of inequality?"

"Not at all. Negotiation is not the absence of power or regularity. Just because something is in constant process doesn't mean it lacks inequality or stability. Order and states of domination are as inherent to negotiation as are change and chaos. Go back to the case of the therapist and her gambling patients. As the therapist interacts with her patients she maintains varying degrees of domination, oppression and exploitation. She controls the group and what it talks about. She decides which patients are getting better and who will be discharged and when. And so, her constant position of control in the negotiations produces a degree of regularity. Patients come in, one after the other, and learn the rhythm of the treatment program. It becomes taken for granted and has a degree of smoothness to it, primarily as a function of its inequality. But, this dominating smoothness constantly requires staff and patients to negotiate a plethora of breakdowns and fractures."

"So," said Ruby, "discursive negotiations tune us into the spontaneous and improvisational dimensions of domination? They show us that order is a play of forces; a play that never really comes to an end, never stops? It's always going, as you say, right and left, up and down, inside and out—right?"

"Exactly, which is why patients (and even therapists) are able to challenge orders, break certain rules, misuse organizational codes and change the practice of treatment even in a state of static domination. Patients come back from a weekend pass having gambled; therapists disagree with one another and undermine the goals of treatment and so on. And so, despite the stability the unit achieves, its daily functioning, in one way or another, is negotiated. As such, the overall organization that emerges is a negotiated order."

Ruby asked, "Would you say, then, that resistance and freedom are necessary to the practice of the medical model? I mean, it seems to me that because the medical model of pathological gambling is based on negotiation, the degree to which patients and therapists act as free and resisting agents becomes central to understanding the very practices by which they are controlled—yes?"

"Exactly," I said. "Patients and therapists do not simply apply or enact the medical model. They negotiate it: they alter it, change it, make modifications, induce difference. In fact, the history of the medical model of gambling only makes sense if the various discourses and social forces involved (from patients and their families to the gambling industry) are conceptualized as free agents who are able to resist and make different the medical model of gambling. Remember what Anselm Strauss explained: even enemies have to negotiate and work together to arrive at their quite discrepant ends."[4]

"So," said Ruby, "actors, as forces in conflict over differences, must negotiate with one another to arrive at their various ends. And these acts of negotiation surrounding the construction and usage of knowledge, you call them discursive negotiations?"

"You've got it. Care, help, love and solidarity, assistance, cooperation, collaboration, teamwork and harmony, they all take place right along side of domination and exploitation. It all bleeds into one another, the good and the bad, there is no clear division. Discursive negotiations attempt to capture this blurring of the lines, the points at which discourses are used to help and hurt at the same time, and the mechanisms by which these processes play themselves out."

"And so you would say that most doctors are not evil incarnate and that most pathological gamblers are not passive lambs?"

"Exactly. I think therapists and patients are much more than these overly simplistic reductions and caricatures. Therapists heal and hurt. Patients manipulate and cooperate. It's as simply complicated as that. The relationship between doctors and patients is certainly asymmetrical, but it's not all domination and resistance. Discourses are always in inter-action having a variety of effects, both good and bad and somewhere in-between. The complexity is further compounded by the fact that the process doesn't stop. The effects of one set of discursive negotiations cross-over and run through another set of negotiations, which then bounce and collide off of discursive negotiations elsewhere. It is out of this process, this multiplicity, this assemblage that discursive social change takes place."

As Ruby and I talked on, I explained to her that my theory and method emerged out of my own negotiations with the texts of Anselm Strauss and Michel Foucault. Foucault's poststructuralist ideas about the relationship between power and knowledge were very influential on my thinking. But, despite his influence, I felt that Foucault's definition of power, while consistent with the general ideas of Strauss and other symbolic interactionists, was, in the end, limited: it defined only one dimension of inter-action. I was interested in inter-action in general and not just power. And so I needed a conceptual framework that could handle the challenges and insights of Foucault, while at the same time being sensitive to the negotiated realities of discursive existence that I was finding in my study. I found my answer in the work of Anselm Strauss. Working things out between Foucault and Strauss, I was able to come up with the beginnings of a theory I now call *discursive interactionism* and a method I call *assemblage*.

Nearing the end of my conversation with Ruby, I said "you know, my problem with these ideas is that they're only fragments of a thought." "Most of life," she responded, "is lived clinging to a fragmented web of incomplete thought. It doesn't matter. Besides, your goal at this point isn't to create a systematic theory or method anyway." "But then what is my goal?" "Be a good student of Foucault, be a good interactionist. Like I said before, your goal is to challenge yourself and others to think differently about the topic of pathological gambling and to create the necessary tools to do that."

My initial conversations with Ruby are in the past now, and yet I remember them vividly. I had stumbled on to what I felt were a number of important ideas about the history of pathological gambling. I spent the next three years working on this study. When I finished it, I gave it to Ruby to read. We negotiated our differences as well as our similarities. We came to our own conclusions. Now I'm interested in what you think.

PART II

Chapter 1

THE BIRTH OF GAMBLING AS A MEDICAL OBJECT OF INVESTIGATION

It All Began as a Negotiated Moment amongst Wider—Radical—Discursive Negotiations Already Taking Place

The moment was a pre-trial hearing held before the honorable José A. Cabranes. The date was 22 September 1983. The location was the United States District Court, Second Circuit. The Second Circuit pre-trial hearing came in the aftermath of an unprecedented move on the part of the prosecution. The prosecution asked Judge Cabranes to reverse centuries of legal tradition and institute a change so radical that only two states had so far adopted it. On 16 May 1983, the prosecution submitted a Brandeis-Brief requesting that the insanity defense be abolished. Judge Cabranes, taken back, stated that the gutsy request was "without parallel in American law . . ." (United States v. Torniero, 570 F. Supp. p.722, 1983). In anxious response, the defense submitted their own brief on 13 June 1983.

The cause for this federal, pre-trial hearing was John Torniero. On 23 September 1982, John Torniero was charged with ten counts of interstate transportation of stolen property. Torniero had worked as a store manager for Michael's Jewelers in New Haven, Connecticut. Over a two year period Torniero repeatedly stole diamonds from his employer and, either by himself or with the help of others, transported the jewels across the Connecticut–New York border. Once in New York, he took the jewelry into an area of New York City known as the "Diamond Exchange" and sold them. To cover himself, Torniero falsified various invoices, inventories and other records. Somewhere during the two year period in question, the owners of Michael's Jewelers hired a private investigator. The investigator figured out Torniero's scheme and had him arrested. Testimony at the trial indicated that Torniero's thievery amounted to roughly $750,000 dollars in loss to Michael's Jewelers.[1]

What made this case so important weren't the charges Torniero was facing. Putting forth a defense of insanity was nothing new. What made this case so controversial, and caused the prosecution to react so strongly, was the line of defense taken by Torniero's attorneys. They argued that Torniero was legally insane at the time of his crimes because he was a pathological gambler. Shortly after his arrest, Torniero was taken to see Dr. Marvin A. Steinberg, a licensed psychologist. After their first session, Steinberg diagnosed Torniero as suffering from the mental disease *pathological gambling*. Being a pathological gambler meant that Torniero was "chronically and progressively unable to resist impulses to gamble" (American Psychiatric Association 1980, p. 291), which meant that he was unable to resist the impulse to steal to keep his gambling going. At the time of the trial, Steinberg was quoted as saying "Due to Mr. Torniero's condition of pathological gambling, he was unable to conform his behavior to the requirements of the law."[2]

There Were Wider—Radical—Discursive Negotiations Taking Place at the Time of Torniero's Case

The reason a defense of insanity based on pathological gambling caused such a stir was because in 1983, unlike alcoholism or drug addiction, the legal aspects of the medical diagnosis of pathological gambling had yet to be worked out in a court of law. With the publication of pathological gambling as a medical disorder in the 1980 edition of the DSM-III (*The Diagnostic and Statistical Manual of Mental Disorders,* 3rd Edition, published by the American Psychiatric Association), at once the problems associated with it changed from vice to disease.

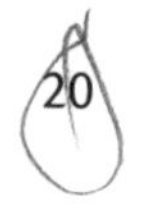

> 312.31 Pathological Gambling
>
> The essential features are a chronic and progressive failure to resist impulses to gamble and gambling behavior that compromises, disrupts, or damages personal, family, or vocational pursuits. . . . Characteristic problems include loss of work due to absences in order to gamble, defaulting on debts and other financial responsibilities, disrupted family relationships, borrowing money from illegal sources, forgery, fraud, embezzlement, and income tax evasion. (American Psychiatric Association 1980, p. 291)

With the publication of the DSM-III, a shift in the discursive history of gambling took place and a new medical problem was born. It didn't matter that pathological gambling was classified as an impulse control disorder and not as an addiction. All that mattered was that it had entered the psychiatric and mental health literature. It had an entirely new status and existence. Under the guiding intellectual support of certain key researchers and clinicians in the field of mental health, pathological gambling emerged as a major challenge to the legal, governmental, economic, political, religious and cultural definitions by which gambling had been previously defined, understood, and treated since the late 1800s. If Torniero had been arrested just three years earlier, in 1979, his defense of insanity would have been impossible. His case would have been just another day in court. Because it took place after 1980, things were different. After 1980, a shift took place. The medical model now stood as a challenge to the legal, thereby challenging our cultural and political conceptions of gambling in courtrooms across America.

An important article during the 1980s cataloging the challenges pathological gambling brought to the legal system was written by the noted gambling law professor I. Nelson Rose. Rose's article was part of a special edition for the *Journal of Gambling Studies,* which was, and still is, the only journal specifically devoted to the topic of pathological gambling. The subject of the special edition was "Compulsive Gambling and the Law." In his article Rose (1988) wrote:

> The idea that compulsive gambling is a disease is in direct conflict with the dominant view in the law that gambling is a vice. Under the traditional view individuals who gamble to excess

> are morally weak and deserving of punishment. The recognition of "pathological gambling" as an official mental disease or disorder by the American Psychiatric Association in 1980 created an irreconcilable contention: American law never punishes an individual for being sick. The conflict can be seen in every area of the law and even between judges sitting in the same courtroom. The most dramatic disputes have been over the insanity defense; but, the disease argument has been raised, sometimes successfully, in other criminal cases, to mitigate sentencing, in attorney disbarments, tax cases, bankruptcies, divorces, personal injury claims, and, most significantly, in claims against casinos. The legal disputes will spread and become even more heated as the disease diagnosis becomes more generally accepted. (P. 240)

During the 1980s, Torniero's case was only one of a number of court cases at the state and federal level challenging the legal definitions of insanity as well as the court's understanding and treatment of pathological gambling and its problems. By 1981 two different defendants had already used pathological gambling as an insanity defense and won. The first was in Torniero's home state of Connecticut (United States v. Lafferty 1983). The second in New Jersey (United States v. Campanaro) (See also Rose 1988). Other court cases were not as successful. In the United States v. Lewellyn case (1983), the defense tried to convince the Eight Circuit Court of Appeals that their client was not guilty of attempting to embezzle $17,000,000 in securities because he suffered from pathological gambling. The court didn't go for it, arguing that a sufficient causal relationship couldn't be established between pathological gambling and criminal activity that "could be considered binding upon the legal system" (Cunnien, 1985, p. 91). In another case, Genevieve Banks tried to counter-sue Resorts International for $75,000 in losses. Banks claimed that Resorts International, who happened to be suing her to recover a $1,000 gambling debt, owed her the money she lost at their casino because she was a diagnosed pathological gambler. Disagreeing with Banks, "the Superior Court of New Jersey granted Resorts' motion for summary judgement and dismissal of the counterclaim on the ground the casino had followed state law in issuing credit" (Rose, 1988, p. 255).

Pathological gambling was also being used to assuage the severity of sentencing in both criminal and civil cases. For example, a Louisiana lawyer who had been convicted of felonies involving "deceit and dishonesty" was given only a two-year suspension because he suffered "from a psychological or emotional disorder consisting of a compulsive or addictive gambling habit or disease" (Rose, 1988, p. 248). Instead of sentencing him to jail, "the court put great weight on the lawyer undergoing medical treatment, attending Gamblers Anonymous, and 'making a sincere effort to rehabilitate himself and to recover from his illness'" (Rose, 1988, p. 248). And, in a civil case, Mr. Milton H. Guillot sued his employer for firing him without notice or explanation. After being fired, Milton "suffered a nervous breakdown, was hospitalized and, after being released, continued to have emotional troubles, including compulsive gambling and heavy drinking. The Louisiana Court of Appeal affirmed an award of partial disability workmen's compensation" (Rose, 1988, p. 253).

Throughout the 1980s and 1990s, the medical discourses of pathological gambling would continue to challenge the judicial system. In each case the definitions of right, responsibility, treatment and punishment were questioned. By reconstructing excessive gambling as an entirely new medical phenomena, the mental health industry birthed a *new* social problem; a new social problem that not only required transformations in law, but extended outward through a web of discursive negotiations crisscrossing any and all of the various fields and formations pertaining to gambling to affect the way Americans think about the problems of gambling. While Torniero's day in court was unprecedented, it was merely one instance, a symptom if you will, of the wider, radical discursive negotiations taking place at the time.

The Compulsive Gambler Suffers from a Disease of the Mind

While the medical model of pathological gambling obtained a position of professional authority in the 1980s, it has been around since the 1940s.

The year was 1943. An article titled "The Gambler: A Misunderstood Neurotic" was published in the journal *Criminal Psychopathology.* The article was written by Edmund Bergler, who, with this publication, marked with ink the beginning of a new history.[3] While 1943 marked the beginning, it wasn't until 1958 that Bergler finally published his classic *The Psychology of Gambling.* It is the book most often cited today as the official starting point of the medical investigation of excessive gambling. In the preface Bergler outlined his view:

> Boiled down, the popular concept of a gambler is that he is a person who wants to make as much money as he can with the least expenditure of time and effort. The unconscious reaction of the average person to the gambler is mixed. Secretly, he admires the gambler when he wins and gloats when he loses, as if to say: "Why should he achieve what ordinary people cannot?" What is never asked is this decisive question: "Does the gambler really *want to win*?" Gambling, in the popular mind, is a dangerous and difficult activity, but one which is none the less *rational.*
>
> Some people object to gambling, but their objections have moral, religious, or social reasons. When the psychology of gamblers is viewed through the psychiatric-psychoanalytic microscope, it becomes clear that the basic problem is precisely that point which is erroneously taken for granted and considered self-evident: the gambler's apparent aim to win. I submit that the gambler is not simply a rational though "weak" individual who is willing to run the risk of failure and moral censure in order to get money the easy way, but a *neurotic with an unconscious wish to lose*. . . .
>
> The purpose of this book is to substantiate, with clinical proof, the theory that the gambler has an unconscious wish to lose—and therefore always loses in the long run. (1958, p. vii)

With the opening pages of his book, Bergler established the framework for the paradigm shift the DSM-III would finally announce. With these pages Bergler makes a full break with the past by redressing the problems of gambling within the new and powerful discourses of medicine and psychiatry. Bergler defines the pathological gambler outside the domain of sin or vice. In fact, he chastises those who still see excessive gambling within the territory of the rational, the conscious, the ego. Pathological gambling and the problems associated with it are manifestations of a sickness, an illness, an error deep within the psyche. Gone are the days, argues Bergler, when the problems of gambling will remain trapped within the rational. Contrary to the popular, albeit facile mentality, the excessive gambler is not simply a racketeer, criminal, malefactor, mobster, or con-artist. The excessive gambler can no longer be viewed within these arcane manifestations of legal and moral myth. These pervasive, fashionable perceptions are merely representations of an otherwise unconscious hostility toward the romantic life of the gambler. A series of discursive negotiations must take place between the psychiatric expert and the rest of society. The judge, the attorney, the police commissioner, the average person on the street, they all must be taught to work through their own unconscious archetypal representations of "the gambler" to learn the "true" nature of this disorder: that is, its medical and psychiatric basis. They must come to understand, with sympathy, the pathological person they are dealing with. They must recognize that the pathological gambler is sick. The pathological gambler suffers from a disease of the mind. The pathological gambler is someone who cannot control himself. He is not a loser or a failure. The job of society, in order to correct these problems, is not to punish. Punishment, explains Bergler, is for the criminal, the gangster, the gambler-racketeer not the sucker gambler, the neurotic, the individual with the unconscious desire to lose. If society is going to provide a solution in an attempt to restore order, then it must be in the form of rehabilitation, clinical treatment, hours spent in the psychiatrist's office or in the insane asylum. We cannot confuse the two, the criminal and the neurotic. Bergler (1958) states: "This book is about the neurotic sucker-gambler, hence about psychopathology. The gambler-racketeer belongs in the realm of criminology, and deserves a separate psychological investigation" (p. viii).

During the 1950s while Bergler was fast at work on the east coast establishing the medical model of pathological gambling, Gamblers Anonymous (GA) was getting its start on the west coast. While GA had several false starts in other parts of the country, it finally came together in Los Angeles, California. The first meeting was held on a Friday, 13 September 1957. GA patterned itself after Alcoholics Anonymous (AA). When AA first started back in 1935, it was opposed to the medical model. It endorsed the medical model several years later, however, to gain credibility within the general public because the medical model argued that alcoholism was a mental illness and not simply a matter of a weak will. GA followed suit and adopted the medical model into its own program: "We, at Gamblers Anonymous, believe our gambling problem is an emotional illness, progressive in nature, which no amount of human will-power can stop or control. We have facts to support this belief" (Gamblers Anonymous 1989, p. 38).

While psychoanalytic treatment and GA existed for pathological gambling during the 1950s and 1960s, it wasn't until the 1970s that pathological gambling gained a greater level of credibility within the larger field of mental health. In the field of mental health, pathological gambling made its first major move toward respectability when Dr. Robert Custer, Director of the Veterans Addiction Recovery Program (Veterans Administration Medical Center, Brecksville, Ohio), established the first in-patient gambling treatment program. Dr. Custer, a psychiatrist who specialized in addiction treatment, was approached by a members of a local GA group who were having trouble with a few of their members who were suffering from severe psychological problems. Working closely with Gamblers Anonymous, Custer and "the Brecksville team established a therapy program. The program was expanded and the first in-patient treatment facility for compulsive gamblers was opened in 1972 . . ." (Rosecrance, 1985a, p. 278). Custer states:

> My associate Alida Glen, Ph.D., and I designed a treatment program patterned after the one we were using to treat alcoholics.
>
> The compulsive gamblers were given individual counseling relating mainly to the control of the gambling urge and on practical problems such as marital strife, their debts, the family's financial needs. In addition to that, there was group therapy, where the gamblers got together and, led by a professional psychiatrist, psychologist, social worker or nurse, discussed with each other the way they had gotten into gambling, the problems it had caused them, their feelings of hopelessness, what they thought was wrong with them, their personality defects. In other words, while counseling dealt with the facts, group therapy dealt with their feelings, giving them a chance to ventilate, and to get some insight into themselves and their compulsion. In addition, there were lectures on the nature of the gambling addiction, so they could get an objective view of themselves and their problems. They also went through relaxation training as a way to deal with their pent-up tensions, pressures and agitation. (Custer and Milt 1985, p. 218)

From 1972 onward, both because of his establishment of the Brecksville program and his burgeoning publications, Custer became one of the leading authorities on pathological gambling in the United States. In fact, his book, *When Luck Runs Out,* published in 1985, is the current bible in the field. With the help of Custer, the Brecksville Gambling Treatment Program became recognized as one of the leading treatment programs in the country. It was also Custer who finally got pathological gambling into the DSM-III.

While the work of Bergler and Custer helped pathological gambling increase in its position of power, it remained throughout the 1970s on the margins of mental health and society in general. The reason it remained on the margins wasn't simply a function of Custer needing more time to campaign. Other factors were at work: primarily the gambling industry and state and federal government. When Bergler was writing, gambling was illegal. When Custer was writing, gambling was fast becoming legalized everywhere. Thus, the 1980 publication of the *DSM-III* not only announced the emergence of an entirely new medical disorder, it also announced a legalized gambling explosion.

When Bergler Was Writing, Gambling Was Illegal, Immoral, and Therefore Wrong

In 1958, when Bergler wrote *The Psychology of Gambling,* gambling was still an illegal activity, except for Las Vegas and a few Catholic churches. Of course people gambled during the 1950s and 1960s—gambling had always been and still remains an important part of United States culture. To the mainstream middle-class of the 1950s and 1960s, however, gambling was a morally and legally illegitimate activity. The fact that gambling was illegitimate had a major discursive effect on the construction of Bergler's text, as well as the position and authority of the medical model for the next twenty-two years.

To illustrate my point, let's return to Bergler's preface. In his preface, Bergler makes a distinction between the gangster-racketeer and the neurotic-sucker, which he believes have nothing in common: "The [neurotic] gambler is *unconsciously* driven to gambling, while the racketeer-gambler *consciously* uses gambling, as he would high-jacking, for his *modus operandi*" (Bergler 1958, p. vii, italics in original). While Bergler distinguished these two types of gamblers, thirty years later articles would be published in journals such as the *Journal of Gambling Studies, The Journal of Forensic Sciences,* and *Clinical Forensic Psychiatry* with titles such as "The Pathological Gambler as Criminal Offender" (Rosenthal & Lorenz, 1992), "Criminal Offenses in Gamblers Anonymous and Hospital Treated Pathological Gamblers" (Blaszczynski & McConaghy, 1994), "Crime, Antisocial Personality and Pathological Gambling" (Blaszczynski, McConaghy, & Frankova, 1989), and "Correlates of Pathological Gambling Propensity in Prison Inmates" (Templer, Kaiser, & Siscoe, 1993). And these articles would make claims such as: "Many personality features characteristic of antisocial personality disorders are reputedly found to be inherent in pathological gamblers . . ." (Blaszczynski & McConaghy, 1994, p. 130).

Our question then is: if in the 1990s there is no real clinical difference between Bergler's sucker and the racketeer (both lie, cheat, write bad checks, steal from their employers, and con family and friends for money to support their habit) why does Bergler maintain such a distinction? The answer? In the 1950s gambling was illegal. Therefore, the discourses of law and religion prevailed. These discourses viewed gambling as a rational activity done with full conscious intent. The only way Bergler could alter these perceptions was to create a discourse that did not encroach upon the disciplinary and legal boundaries of the court or criminal justice system. Bergler (1958) makes the boundary clear: "This book is about the neurotic-gambler, hence about psychopathology. The gambler-racketeer belongs in the realm of criminology . . ." (p. viii). In the 1950s, anyone caught gambling would immediately be viewed as a criminal. Bergler would have had little success convincing politicians or judges that the pathological gambler standing before them had unconsciously embezzled $500,000 dollars because he had a infantile fantasy to destroy his life and therefore needed a year of psychoanalysis and GA, not prison.

Bergler thought that if people would just take a peek through the microscope of medicine they would see the criminal before them transform into a person with a mental illness: "Some people object to gambling, but their objections have moral, religious, or social reasons. When the psychology of gamblers is viewed through the psychiatric-psychoanalytic microscope, it becomes clear that the basic problem is precisely that point which is erroneously taken for granted and considered self-evident: the gambler's apparent aim to win" (1958 p. vii). But Bergler was not dumb. He knew the change in perception he was arguing for would have a limited range of effect. He therefore acquiesced by setting up a discursive boundary between the neurotic and the criminal. As long as neurotics are caught gambling, they remain criminals. But for those neurotics lucky enough to make it into Bergler's office, they are, in the eyes of medicine, not deserving of punishment but treatment. If these same neurotics were arrested by the police leaving Bergler's office, they would once again be criminals.

The boundaries Bergler constructed between the court room and the clinical couch, between the medical profession and criminal justice system, between the neurotic and the criminal, between the pathological gambler and the rest of society would remain "true" for the next twenty two years. And it would have stayed that way if not for the third wave of gambling legalization.

In 1963, the Third Wave of Gambling Legalization Began

In 1963 the third wave of legalized gambling began its sweep across the United States. It started with New Hampshire, which legalized the first state lottery since the 1890s.[4] New Jersey, New York and Massachusetts were quick to follow. By the early 1990s lotteries existed in over thirty-seven states, and twenty-three states had some form of state sponsored gambling such as casinos, riverboats, dog tracks, horse tracks, off-track sports betting or bingo parlors. The annual revenue from gambling during the 1990s was more than the movie, book, record, park and arcade industries combined (Hirshy, 1994). In fact, in 1993 alone, Americans bet a staggering $400 billion dollars on legalized gambling—"a figure that grew at an average annual rate of almost 15 percent a year between 1992 and 1994" (Goodman, 1995, p. 2). Looking toward the year 2000, Phil Sartre, President of Harrah's Casinos, one of the world's largest casino companies, estimated that "ninety-five percent of all Americans will most likely live in a state with legal casino entertainment" (Goodman 1995, p. 3).

But why the change? Why did gambling all of a sudden become legalized again? And why so fast? Was it because the general public wanted it? It doesn't seem to be the case. Goodman (1995) states:

> One of the most surprising findings of our research is that we didn't come across a single popularly based organization that

> lobbies for more gambling. Many other government prohibitions—such as laws against the smoking of marijuana—have inspired popular legalization movements. But not gambling. In fact, when given the chance to make its views known, the public usually rejects gambling. . . .
>
> So if it's not the public, who is behind the push for more gambling opportunities? Two parties are almost entirely responsible: legislators in search of easy answers to tough economic problems, and the gambling industry itself. (P. x)

Prior to 1963, the gambling industry was certainly interested in expanding its business. But, it had to wait for government to make the first move. During the 1970s and 1980s, even though state lotteries were being legalized everywhere, they weren't generating the profits expected. It was at that point that the gambling industry was called upon to help. They knew what games people liked and how to market them. It was only a matter of time, then, before most politicians became convinced that gambling was the way to save their cities and states from financial ruin. Once the doors to legalized gambling were opened, the gambling industry's campaign could not be stopped. The campaign followed two basic steps: first a set of "pro-gambling" discourses were constructed, then these discourses were used to negotiate with others both to gain support and argue against detractors.

Creating a Discourse

The first goal in the campaign was to create a discourse by which an argument for legalized gambling could be made. This discourse had to argue from a position that could overcome the discourses of religion, culture and law still in circulation. The discourse chosen was one based on a combination of economic policy and "scientific" research. The arguments were put forth succinctly: your state, city or town is in economic trouble, you have people out of work, your standard of living has decreased, and you have no other real options available. If you legalize gambling, jobs will be created, money will be given to the schools, your town's economic recession will be lifted, the standard of living will increase, people from out of state will come in to gamble; the restaurants, hotels, malls, bars, and stores in your area will make money, and everyone will be happy. We guarantee it.

From the beginning, the business people and local community leaders in the more economically depressed areas of the country were sold. Others, not nearly as bad off, were suspicious. The majority, who were indeed struggling but were not sure what to do, were somewhere in the middle. As Mayor Robert Markle of Springfield, Massachusetts stated: "The city of Springfield had its back to the wall . . . This would not be my first choice, but we don't seem to have a lot of choices right now" (Goodman 1995, p. viii). During the 1980s, as economic decline spread outward into more and more cities, negotiations increasingly turned in the direction of legalized gambling.

To construct their discourses of promise, the gambling industry (or the private firms it hired) conducted numerous "scientific" studies to examine the problems of economic decline, as well as the ways in which legalizing gambling could counteract these problems. In all of these studies, the same basic assumption was made: "With so much untapped demand for gambling in the country, and with so little gambling available, the economic results of expansion could not help but be positive" (Goodman 1995, p. 65). It was obvious, so they argued, that gambling "would create hundreds of millions of dollars in additional public revenues and thousands of new private-sector jobs" (Goodman 1995, p. 65). Because the research was done primarily by the gambling industry itself, or some hired research group, seldom were the problems that came with legalized gambling mentioned. Studies did not directly address the problems of addiction, crime, or its long-term economic consequences. Goodman (1995) elaborates:

> While some states have commissioned expensive research, ostensibly designed as an objective aid to policy makers, the research was in fact often prepared just to support the positions of those who had already decided in favor of gambling expansion. For example, one study prepared for the state of Connecticut at a cost of nearly a quarter of a million dollars, by Christiansen/Cummings Associates, a New York research firm with close ties to the gambling industry, concluded that the state's "mature" and sometimes declining gambling operations would soon face competition from a local tribal casino and new

> gambling ventures in other states. "Faced with this rather bleak future," said consultants, "the state of Connecticut *must* consider new gambling options" (their emphasis).
>
> The report made no significant reference to the public and private costs of such "must" options other than to note that compulsive gambling was a problem and that a higher percentage of the state's population were likely to become compulsive gamblers, and then to make cursory mention that the state should take steps to deal with this problem. Nonetheless, the study recommended that Connecticut provide more enticing gambling opportunities, more lottery advertising, and more incentives for lottery agents to sell more tickets. (Pp. 65–66)

Goodman makes it clear that unstated political biases clearly controlled the outcome of "state sponsored" research. Goodman and his associates explored fourteen studies done for various state and local areas. Goodman (1995) concluded that, of the fourteen studies, ten were unbalanced or mostly unbalanced in their ability to objectively describe "the real public and private benefits and costs to a community or state" (p. 66), and only one was fairminded and balanced in its presentation of the "facts."

Negotiating with Others

Once the discourses were researched and constructed, the next step was to convince everyone. Some of the most important positions involved in the negotiations included local and state level businesses, community and religious leaders, the education system—which is where most of the money goes—the television and print media, and the middle and working classes. An example of how the process of negotiation works comes from the attempt to legalize riverboat gambling in Ohio.[5]

During the 1996 election year, pro-gambling business, with the help of certain lawyers, tried to pass a bill to legalize limited riverboat gambling. It was called *Issue One*. Three months before the vote I was in Cleveland with some friends. While we were drinking our coffee a man approached us. He asked us if we would like to sign a petition in support of riverboat gambling. He explained to us the advantages of legalizing gambling. "What will Ohio win if riverboat casinos are introduced?" we asked. "Benefits include $1.28 billion in annual onsite gambling and non-gambling spending, annual operational expenditures of $172.8 million on Ohio goods and services, and 21,175 new permanent jobs. For a tax of 20 percent on all casino revenues that remain after winnings are paid to participants, the state will receive $232.2 million annually. In addition, another $38.1 million in other taxes, including those on property, food and beverages and alcohol, will be collected. Eighty percent of the $232.2 million in riverboat casino tax revenues, or about $186 million will be earmarked for Ohio public schools" (Yes on Issue 1 Committee 1996, p. 1). Picking up his clip board he said: "So, would you like to sign my petition?"

I won't tell you if we signed his petition or not, but I did ask him if he had any other information beyond what he had initially provided. He explained that he worked for a local polling company which had been hired to put the issue on the upcoming ballet. Frustrated with my persistent questioning, he finally said he could care less about the issue. In fact, he was completely ignorant about the issue other than the memorized speech he had given me. I asked him for his business card.

The next week I made a few phone calls to find out who had contacted his agency to go out and do the polling. It was pro-gambling business people—capitalism working at the grass roots level. People were signing the petition with little to no knowledge about the issue. And they were often signing, as I watched, just so the man would go away. They wanted to enjoy their meals in peace. Obviously the tactic worked, three months later the issue was on the 1996 Ohio ballot.

And So Gambling Was Legalized

And so, between the years of 1963 and 1998, gambling was legalized throughout most of the United States. The process was slow at first but picked up speed as one state after another jumped on board. As the number of states legalizing gambling increased, their pro-gambling discourses began to intersect, cross-over and build off of one another, like a disease spreading out across the country, creating a nation-wide epidemic. These interactions were carried through the radio waves. They moved from computer to computer. They crossed through the television and its commercials. They fell upon the ears of those listening or watching the evening news. They leaped from one business person to the next while discussing gambling profits. They happened as friends and family, visiting from one state to the next, talked about the joys of playing the lottery. They took place when a sports star said "I'm going to Las Vegas after the Super Bowl." They moved outward when a community leader endorsed a new casino. And finally, they gained legislative support as politician after politician wrote them into bills. As this process took place, in and between, through and across, above and below all of the various interactions happening across the country, the majority of people in the United States began to move away from the dominating influence of the moral and legal texts. During the course of these interactions, there were those who remained opposed to gambling. Regardless, as the wave of gambling legitimation crossed from city to city, state to state, moving outwardly inward through all of the various negotiated fields of discursive relations, the dominant view began to move in the direction of legitimization and legalization. High and low, within, between and across every level, old ways of understanding gambling broke down until gambling finally became legitimate and legal. A radical break with the past took place. The larger field of discursive relations concerning gambling changed.

Emergent from this change were new gambling objects of investigation, new concepts and vocabularies, new theories, and new voices of authority. The new discourses and concepts arrived in the form of gambling business theory. The gambler (the gamer) became a rational consumer who was able to make decisions about where and when to gamble. The gambler was a person who enjoyed the activity of gambling strictly for the purposes of recreation and pleasure. The gambler knew how much he or she had available for gambling and knew when too much money had been spent. The voices of authority became the gambling industry and government. The goal and objective of the gambling industry was to provide the gambling consumer with a wide variety of gambling activities and to see gambling legalized in as many states as possible; not because it wanted to create an opiate for the masses, but because it desired, as with any business, to make a profit. The goal of the gambling industry was to generate revenue. Their goal was to minimize cost, maximize output, control quality. They distributed their product, reinvested part of their profits in the company, took the other part home. Businesses competed with others. Casinos, horse tracks, and river boats attempted to put their opponents out of business, beat them in price, overcome them in quantity, and without sacrificing a relative level of quality. Competition between gambling businesses helped to build the economy. It provided jobs and money for education. It increased the standard of living and helped to promote the overall economy. Gambling became entertainment. Las Vegas became a place to take the family on vacation and the lottery became something even grandma played on the weekend. The campaigns of state and city governments and their gambling industry counterparts had been, on the whole, incredibly successful. So what was the problem?

The Establishment of the Medical Model

The primary problem during the 1980s and 1990s was that, once the third wave of gambling legalization took off, the boundaries Bergler had temporarily constructed between the court room and the clinical couch, between the medical profession and the criminal justice system, between the neurotic and the criminal, between the pathological gambler and the rest of society, collapsed. There was no longer a clear division between the excessive gambler showing up for in-patient treatment and the excessive gambler showing up for court. Once gambling became legalized, the criminal justice system fell in power, position, and authority. The proper political solutions to the problems of gambling—as evidenced by Torniero's trial—were no longer clear. The publication of the DSM-III, therefore, not only marked the official emergence of the medical model, it more importantly signaled that a precedent had been set by the process of legalization itself. Legalization challenged the very foundations of law. If everyone was now allowed to gamble, then the legal discourses no longer maintained complete jurisdiction. Pathological gambling, once easily classified as a crime, now appeared complex.

But the courts, as well as the rest of society, didn't know how to deal with the new complexities. Legalization left the criminal justice system without the necessary tools to deal with the problems they were now facing. As with alcohol, drugs, and other various potential vices, availability always multiplies the number of people who fall prey to the trappings of addiction. Once casinos and lotteries started popping up all over the country, it was understandable that in-patient addiction treatment facilities, local police departments, and the criminal justice system would experience increases in gambling related problems (e.g., crime, credit card fraud, checking and banking scandals, family problems, loss of jobs, psychological breakdown, bankruptcies, inability to pay debts to casinos and bookies, and so on). Of the total population, the people hit hardest by the problems of pathological gambler were the middle-class.

Rosecrance (1985a) explains:

> Traditionally, gambling has been tacitly accepted by the working and upper classes (Downes, 1976; Newman, 1972). In contrast, serious and sustained gambling has not been a typical pattern of behavior in the middle-class (Newman, 1968). Until recently, then, middle-class individuals had relatively limited personal or associative experience with gambling and its possible consequences. Lacking such experience, many middle-class gamblers are relatively unprepared for the psychological pressures of losing and winning (Berry, 1968; Beyer, 1978; Martinez and LaFranchi, 1969; Newman, 1975). On the one hand, they have not learned a repertoire of techniques for dealing with the periodic losses that are an integral part of sustained gambling. On the other hand, a large win or "big score" early in the gambling career of a middle-class participant can lead to unrealistic and unfulfilled expectations of continued winnings. The middle-class gambler often has access to lines of credit and other sources of funds that are unavailable to lower-class gamblers. Such resources allow gambling to continue to the point where large debts may threaten the middle-class gambler's financial and social status. (Pp. 280–281)

Because the middle-class, during the 1980s, had access to enormous lines of credit and because they generally lacked the skills necessary to handle the losing phases of gambling, and because gambling fulfills so many other unmet social and psychological needs (e.g., boredom with work and life, retirement, failed marriages, problems with impulsivity and attention deficit, frustration in school, economic depression), pathological gambling began to reach epidemic proportions. Statistics during the 1980s and 1990s reported that about 3.4 percent of the population was addicted to gambling (e.g., Volberg 1994; Volberg and Steadman 1988). In fact, "according to a 1994 Harrah's Casinos survey, the number of American households playing at casinos doubled from 46 million to 92 million between 1990 and 1993, with more than three-quarters of the increase, roughly 35 million households, at new casinos outside of Nevada and New Jersey" (Goodman, 1995, p. 43). Because of these radical increases in gambling, researchers estimated that roughly 9.3 million adults and 1.3 million teenagers had developed some form of gambling problem (Goodman, 1995, p. 43).

It was at the point of recognizing that pathological gambling was fast becoming a social problem that the medical model moved from its position of marginal status to a relatively central position in the debate over how best to now define, understand, and treat the problems of gambling. But why the medical model? Why not other ways of thinking about pathological gambling?

In the aftermath of rapid legalization, there were two primary reasons why the medical model obtained its position of centrality. First of all, while politicians, economists, entrepreneurs, gambling councils, addiction treatment facilities, and the general public became increasingly aware of the problems of gambling, social scientists seemed completely ignorant of the issue. During the early 1980s, other than a handful of psychiatrists, psychologists, addiction treatment counselors, and recovering people, nobody else really did any research on the problems of pathological gambling. The same is true today. Even though pathological gambling affects as many lives as most of the other major mental illnesses, and even though it is almost as devastating as drug addiction and alcoholism, it remains a disorder without disciplinary or professional support, without funding, and without substantial research or theory. In light of the paucity of concern, adherents of the medical model had little difficulty establishing themselves as a dominant discursive force.

Second, and more importantly, we live in a society where social problems on the whole (e.g., crime, welfare, addiction) are defined as issues of health care (Foucault 1965, 1979; Turner 1987; Zola 1972). The United States is a hyper-individualistic, psychologically-oriented, medicalized society that fails to appreciate the larger and smaller social context in which most of its major problems emerge (Conrad & Schneider 1980). In fact, most social scientists wait until medicine defines something as a problem before they recognize it. Because we live in a highly medicalized society, the most likely discourse to fill the gaps left by the criminal justice system, religion, and the social sciences was the medical model. During the early 1980s no other discourse held the level of power it did.

Sheila Blume (1987), one of the leading clinicians and researchers in the field of gambling studies, explains:

> The medical model encourages the development and financial support of resources to help pathological gamblers and their families, and to educate health care providers in identification, intervention, treatment and referral. . . . It also provides a framework for enlightened public policy in the regulation of the gambling industry, and for rational approaches to social and legal problems related to the disease. Gamblers Anonymous, a fellowship founded in 1957 on the same principles as Alcoholics Anonymous, has found the disease concept of compulsive gambling a helpful factor in recovery. (Gamblers Anonymous, 1984, p. 244)

As suggested by Blume, the main reason why the medical model became a dominant discourse on pathological gambling is because no other discourse—other than the legal—could provide the same level of social, cultural, personal, political or economic authority, position or power. Unless something better came along—with "better" defined not as an advancement in science but as an advancement in politics and cultural rhetoric—it would remain the model of choice. And why wouldn't it? What other discourse today, besides the economic, has the potential to free someone from criminal sentencing, loosen cultural stigma, gain the backing of third-party insurance, and provide the basis for obtainable political change? Bottom line, "the 'medical model' is an approach designed to produce change" (Blume 1987, p. 239), and the "disease concept of pathological gambling like the disease concept of alcoholism provides a personally and socially useful approach" (Blume 1987, p. 243).

The Challenges of Medicalization: Is the Gambler Responsible or Not?

While the medical model helped solve a number of problems left open by the legal system, it was not without its own set of difficulties. It challenged our society's fundamental definitions of right and responsibility, punishment and rehabilitation. Before the publication of the DSM-III, there was no controversy. Gambling was a crime. You punished the gambler, pure and simple. There was no need for rehabilitation. But after the DSM-III, it was all open for question. A new tension was born. Law professor, I. Nelson Rose (1988) summarized this tension as follows:

> Law trails society. Changes occurring in the social order in America inevitably lead to conflicts and eventually to changes in the law. The changes that are taking place in contemporary society in the way we view gambling give us a unique opportunity to observe this slow and painful process at work.
>
> The most dramatic confrontations between the old and the new are being fought out to determine basic notions of justice, punishment, and responsibility. There is no middle ground, no way to compromise, between the opposing views: in a criminal case the particular defendant is either acting out of free will and is therefore liable for his actions, or is ill and cannot be held responsible. Guilty or innocent. The standards of punishment follow: punish or rehabilitate. (P. 257)

Given the tension between the legal and the medical at the time of Torniero's trial—as well as throughout the 1980s and 1990s—a number of important questions emerged. Can pathological gambling really be both a disease and a crime? And, if so, are pathological gamblers responsible for their gambling debts? Are they guilty of their crimes? Are they accountable to their families, to their employers, to their friends? Can you send someone to jail for suffering from a disease? And what about government and big business? If government and big business are the primary dealers of the gambling drug, then aren't they responsible for addicting the United States population to gambling? And what are we to do then, send everyone to treatment? And what about the rest of society? Should we enact a prohibition on the majority just to protect a minority? Is gambling really bad for everyone, or is it a disease that only a small percentage suffer from?

The major players in the field of gambling took sides on these questions. On one side of the debate you had government, business, the gambling industry and the criminal justice system who argued that gamblers are rational, capitalistic creatures who—because they gamble with conscious control—are primarily responsible for their actions and their consequences. On the other side of the debate, which was comprised of the field of gambling studies, Gamblers Anonymous, the gambling counsels and the field of addiction treatment, you had people arguing that pathological gamblers suffer from an illness, a disease of the mind, and therefore require compassion and treatment.

Of course, neither side completely ignored the other. Most of those who argued for punishment understood the need for treatment, and most of those who argued for treatment understood the need for punishment. Nevertheless, despite such a sophisticated awareness on the part of the majority of discursive actors involved in the making of pathological gambling, few stood in the middle politically, economically, theoretically or clinically. In fact, so important were the differences between these two perspectives that the history of pathological gambling and its medicalization since the 1980s can be defined by their quarrel. It is to this history, therefore, and the various reasons for it, that the rest of this study will be devoted.

Because Torniero's pre-trial hearing represents, both historically and metaphorically, the major arguments surrounding the organizing practice of pathological gambling and its medicalization, our movement through this study will follow the natural progress of the trial itself, with a twist. We start with an introduction to the court case (chapter two), followed by an analysis of the defense (chapters three through six) and then prosecution (chapters seven through nine) and then the important discursive actors in support of one side or the other (chapters ten through twelve). We end with the decision of the judge himself (chapter thirteen) deciding how the medical and the legal models should be resolved. The book closes with an epilogue which provides a rather exhaustive framework for the future of gambling research, treatment, education and policy.

practice developed by the social sciences, and adopted by the institutions of social control—such as the prison and the education system—to get at the underlying "truth" about individuals.

In the courtroom—which, for this study, acts as the symbolic arena for the arguments taking place in our larger society regarding the two main approaches to understanding gambling; that is, the legal and the medical—neither culpability nor punishment can be determined without the necessary information about the crime. Our understanding of the legal examination process—and, consequently the larger negotiations taking place in the rest of society—is therefore predicated on five important observations.

1. The examination process is heavily influenced by discourse. While the examination process is a technique for getting at the "truth" about the pathological gambler, as a practice it is only method. What actually determines the end result of the examination is the discourse chosen to guide and interpret its results. For example, I could examine the problems of pathological gambling from a number of different discursive perspectives. I could examine pathological gambling from a sociological perspective, a feminist perspective, a historical perspective, or an economic perspective. In each of these instances, even if the examination process followed a similar method, the different discourses would cause me to ask different questions, pursue different avenues of investigation, focus on different key words or phrases, and make different sets of interpretations. As we will see throughout this study, a medical examination is interested in the patient's presenting symptoms and the underlying disease causing them. A sociological examination, in contrast, is interested in the points of conflict emerging, and the social relations involved in constructing and dealing with the problem. Because the examination process is so embedded within discourse, the discourses chosen to guide the process become crucial. At its most basic, this is what was at stake in the Torniero trial: Which discourse should be used to guide the court's criminal examination, the medical or the legal?

2. The examination process is influenced by social context. While the construction and usage of the exam is heavily influenced by discourse, it is also a function of the social context in which it is generally used. In the courtroom, the examination process follows very specific rules. In a typical criminal case, even when the law itself is on trial, the examination starts with the opening remarks. The prosecution goes first, followed by the defense. Once done, the prosecution engages in its examination of the evi-

dence. Witnesses and experts are brought in to testify and so on. After each witness has been examined by the prosecution, the defense is allowed a cross-examination, to which the prosecution can respond, followed, again, by the defense. This process continues until the prosecution rests. The examination then changes sides. It is now the defense's turn. They follow the same basic pattern as the prosecution, with the prosecution providing cross-examination when necessary. Once the defense has rested, concluding remarks are made. The prosecution goes first followed by the defense. Upon conclusion of the closing remarks, the examination process is completed and decisions about culpability and punishment are made by the court.

The construction of the legal exam affects the "uncovering of truth" in several ways. First, it lacks the level of personal intimacy and trust established between a doctor and patient in a medical examination. In contrast to these more intimate environments, the legal examination is cold and very public. The process of the legal exam is also very rigid. It is not open ended. Witnesses are not free to say what they want. People talk one person at a time. The judge is able to overrule any statements felt to be unrelated to the goal of the examination, and witnesses are held accountable for everything they say. They can't make a mistake and change their mind later without fear of being misrepresented. Most importantly, everybody is trying to "trip" the other person up. The goal is not to get to the "truth." The goal is to sell your "truth" over your opponent's "truth" in order to win the case. Thus, the context of the legal exam plays an important role. It is easy to see how the "truth" about a case can get lost, and that who wins doesn't necessarily have anything to do with who is right. It is a heavily-controlled, highly-rationalized and formal forum where discursive negotiations can be quite volatile and destructive.

3. Understanding the negotiated aspects of the legal exam not only requires us to explore thoroughly the courtroom itself, but also the contexts within which the courtroom is situated. In other words, the processes of negotiated examination are always already situated within a series of social contexts which are, themselves, always already decentered onto other negotiations and other contexts.

In Torniero's case, the defense lawyers want to keep Torniero out of jail. They decenter their examination onto a series of already existing discursive negotiations taking place within the field of gambling studies, gambling treatment, and the gambling councils. They know a social movement is under way. Their negotiations lean up against the medical model to make their argument, to conduct their examination. The medical model's constructed object of investigation is a diseased pathological gambler. The "truth" revealed by the medical exam is an individual who is sick and in need of treatment. Decentering the medical discourses onto the social practices of the criminal justice system, Torniero's lawyers draw the medical discourses into their negotiations with the prosecution in order to influence the exam process of the courtroom. They are negotiating a nonlegal (clinical) discourse into a legal examination process. This causes friction. It challenges the very process of legal examination itself by calling into question the end results of the legal exam. The legal exam is to arrive at two conclusions: is the person guilty, and, if so, what is the appropriate punishment? The medical discourses have an alternative end goal. The medical exam wants to determine what is medically wrong with the individual and what is the best way to rehabilitate the individual. Because the discourses driving the medical and legal exam are different, medical care is set in opposition to legal responsibility, and medical rehabilitation is set against legal punishment. Given the conflict and contradiction between these two opposing positions, one will have to give way to the other and one will take the dominant role in the legal process. These are the issues at stake in the Torniero case.

4. Like confession, the exam is an exchange of forces and not a one-sided application that moves from an institution or expert onto the receiving individual or from an individual onto herself. According to Foucault, the examination allows the examiner to remain hidden while the examined is forced into visibility:

> In discipline it is the subjects who have to be seen. Their visibility assures the hold of power that is exercised over them. It is the fact of being constantly seen, of being able always to be seen, that maintains the disciplined individual in his subjection. And the examination is the technique by which power, instead of emitting the signs of its potency,instead of imposing its mark on its subjects, holds them in mechanisms of objectification. (Foucault 1979, p. 187)

What makes institutional examination so powerful is the degree to which it is taken for granted. Those within the institutions of social control forget, or never become aware of, the discourses guiding their process of examination. It isn't until someone with enough power or position challenges these practices that the basis for them becomes evident. Until lawyers challenged the legal examination, gamblers were seen as criminals. By offering an alternative discursive practice of examination and by challenging the legal with the medical, lawyers were able to alter the legal exam; which altered the "truth" about gambling related crime; which altered the way pathological gamblers are cared for. Thus, instead of seeing the exam as so one-sided, it is better to conceptualize it as a process of negotiation where the information "revealed," as well as "hidden," emerges out of the give-and-take inter-actions between the examiner and the examined. The examiner asks certain questions, but the examined must choose to answer. Through this examination process of inter-action, the discursive activities of coercion, manipulation, clarification, intimidation, misrepresentation, persuasion, elucidation and illumination are all at work. Because the examination is negotiated, while the institutions of social control depend upon remaining hidden in order to enforce their position, as in the case of controlling those who will not conform to mainstream morality, the pathological gambler and others, using whatever level of power, authority or position they have, are always challenging and opposing, accepting and denying, giving in to and breaking away from the examination process itself. Even in primary organizations such as the criminal justice system, precedent can reveal, bring to light, the discursive practices dominating the legal exam.

In Torniero's case, the defense and their witnesses negotiate the examination process to convince the judge to think a certain way. The prosecution negotiates with their witness to provide an alternative perspective. In the cross-examination, again, negotiation takes place as witnesses for the defense struggle against the lawyers of the prosecution and vice versa. It is a game of give-and-take.

So important is the negotiated nature of examination that the practice also takes place within the examined individuals themselves. When the individual examines herself, she is playing a game of give-and-take, a game of persuasion where information is hidden, revealed, distorted, made accurate and interpreted according to the situation at hand or the particular need. We often call the act of negotiated self examination the art of self persuasion, but it is not only a matter of truth versus lie. It is fundamental to the very definitions of self that we construct. The individual is acting as both examiner and the examined. In this dual role it becomes a game of discourses chosen and actions intended. These discourses are then believed in, taken for "truth," and argued for in the face of others. In Torniero's case, the lawyers pick their positions. The defense believes in the medical model because they are helping their client. The prosecution disagrees with the medical model because they want to put an end to the insanity defense. Torniero doesn't want to go to jail. After his interview with his psychologist, he more than likely comes to believe that he is not a criminal but a pathological gambler. He suffers from a disease. He now finally understands himself. He wants his lawyers to help him, now that he has found the "truth" about himself. The same process happens with the judge. The pre-trial judge presiding over the case knows the job of the lawyers is to present a one-sided case. The judge therefore has to work through the arguments of both the prosecution and the defense to arrive at a decision. Somewhere amongst the various arguments presented are the "facts" of the case. The judge has his biases as well. He leans toward one side or the other, regardless of his objectivity. He must struggle to deal with his own passions. All of these negotiations are taking place. And yet, in the end, it doesn't matter who is right or who is wrong. A decision is made, and action is taken as a result.

5. Putting all of these parts together, a thorough understanding of the examination comprises analysis of a) the discourses used, b) the social context in which the examination is taking place, c) the structure of the exam itself, d) the larger and smaller contexts and negotiations within which the exam is taking place, and e) the intentions, desired outcomes, and various inter-actions taking place between the actors involved. The exam is therefore neither a thing nor a simple singular action. It is better to conceptualize it as a point of intersection between a series of various processes, which, through their combined effect, result in helping institutions of social control make decisions about how best to care for a given social problem.

The Case of John Torniero

In the first set of negotiations over culpability, two important issues had to be resolved in Torniero's pre-trial hearing. First, the judge had to determine if pathological gambling was a severe enough disease to meet the criteria of the American Law Institute (ALI) test. Second, he had to determine if there was sufficient evidence to warrant a causal link between pathological gambling and criminal behavior. If the judge said "yes" to these issues, then the defense could present expert psychiatric and psychological testimony at the criminal trial on behalf of the insanity defense. If not, the defense would have to argue their case without the usage of expert testimony or reference to insanity or pathological gambling.

Of the various legal tests of insanity available, the ALI test is the most widely adopted at both the state and federal level, and was therefore used in Torniero's pre-trial hearing. The ALI test is a modification of the former test for insanity, the *M'Naghten Rule*. The M'Naghten Rule was established in England in 1843 and quickly became the standard rule in the United States as well. The M'Naghten Rule states that a person is not responsible for criminal acts "if as a result of mental disease of defect he did not understand what he did or that it was wrong, or if he was under a delusion (but not otherwise insane) which, if true, would have provided a good defense" (Gifis 1991, p. 241).

Concerned that a number of important limitations existed with the M'Naghten Rule, the drafters of the Model Penal Code during the 1950s made three important modifications to it and came up with the ALI test. The first modification they made was to substitute the concept of *appreciation* "for that of *cognitive understanding* in the definition of insanity, thus apparently introducing an effective, more emotional, more personalized approach for evaluating the nature of a defendant's knowledge or understanding" (Insanity Defense Work Group 1983, p. 682, italics mine). Second, the group decided that the ALI test should not require the insane person to lack complete appreciation for her behavior, only a "substantial lack of capacity." Third, they decided that the ALI test, like the *Irresistible Impulse Test* should incorporate a "volitional approach to insanity." The volitional prong adds an independent criteria, "the defendant's ability (or inability) to control his actions" (Insanity Defense Work Group 1983, p. 682). As a result of these changes, the ALI test created a new definition of legal insanity: "A person is not responsible for criminal conduct if at the time of such conduct as a result of mental disease or defect he lacks substantial capacity either to appreciate the criminality of his conduct or to conform his conduct to the requirements of law" (Gifis 1991, p. 241).

There was a problem, however, with the ALI test. At the time of Torniero's trial, the ALI test did not list which psychiatric diagnoses were severe enough to be labeled as mental diseases or defects for the purposes of the law. In an attempt to be flexible, the ALI test left it up to the court to decide. Since all of the DSM diagnoses are defined as diseases of the mind, all of them are potentially open for use in an insanity defense. This presented a major problem to the criminal justice system. They had to contend between two very different definitions of insanity: the medical and the legal. The construction, usage, and desired outcomes of these two definitions are very different. The legal system relies upon the insanity plea to help those few individuals who are insane from being wrongfully punished. The field of mental health uses the concept of insanity to claim treatment and research domain over various constellations of problems. The particular balance established between the legal and the medical would, therefore, reveal the professional and institutional politics involved in deciding to what extent a pathological gambler is legally and medically insane. One of these definitions would prevail. In the balance weighed decisions about rights and responsibility, punishment and rehabilitation. In the 1950s, Bergler's model had no impact on the criminal justice system. The disciplinary boundaries were fixed. In a court of law the pathological gambler was a rational criminal. Once the DSM-III was published it all changed. Now the medical was encroaching on the legal. Through other court cases it had already been decided nationally that alcoholism and drug addiction did not meet ALI criteria for legal insanity.[1] The issue of pathological gambling had yet to be determined.

Chapter 3

CONSTRUCTING THE GAMBLING SUBJECT: VIEWS FROM WITHIN THE MEDICAL MODEL

In 1996 an article was published in the American journal *Pharmacogenetics*. Its title read: "A Study of the Dopamine D_2 Receptor Gene in Pathological Gambling." With this article by Comings and colleagues an entirely new medical disorder was empirically validated. Pathological gambling had been recognized for 16 years as a major mental disease of the mind: it had been included in the 1980 publication of DSM-III, and research had been done in the areas of neuropsychology, cognitive-behaviorism, and psychophysiology (e.g., Blaszczynski, McConaghy and Winter 1986; Blanco, Orensanz-Munoz, Blanco-Jerez, and Saiz-Ruiz 1996; Blaszczynski and Silove 1995; Carlton and Manowitz 1992; Rugle and Melamed 1993; Rugle 1993). While all this work had been accomplished, the field still lacked its most important empirical backing, a gene. Now they had it. The medical model of pathological gambling had finally secured its turf (Conrad and Schneider 1980, p. 266).

Before we turn our attention to the arguments of Torniero's defense, I think it is important that we have a better sense of just exactly what the medical model of pathological gambling is. The goal of this chapter is to explore—critically—the discursive strategies used by researchers to understand exactly how the medical model is applied to this phenomena. Examining the discursive strategies used by these researchers is important because it explains how pathological gambling was made into a medical object of investigation and the linguistic slight of hand needed to carry out this work.

What Exactly Is the Medical Model?

Our history of the medicalization of gambling requires, at the very least, a tentative definition of the term "medical model," because it is by and through this concept that we pull together an otherwise diverse set of theories, concepts, and ideas to argue that, historically, the medical model has influenced the way we think and care about excessive gambling and its problems. I will use Conrad and Schneider's definition as it is found in their influential work *Deviance and Medicalization: From Badness to Sickness* (1980). I use this definition because it allows us to define the medical model as a *process* whereby the deviant activity of excessive gambling is medicalized to gain political, economic and cultural control over what has become a major social problem. Conrad and Schneider (1980) define the medical model as follows:

> There are numerous definitions of "the medical model." In this book we adopt a broad and pragmatic definition: the medical model of deviance locates the sources of deviant behavior within the individual, postulating a physiological, constitutional, organic, or, occasionally, psychogenic agent or condition that is assumed to cause the behavioral deviance. The medical model of deviance usually, although not always, mandates intervention by medical personnel with medical means as treatment for the "illness." (P. 35)

Note the rumors spread by this definition. Deviance is found in the organs, the genes, the brain, biological codes. The purpose of the medical definition is to reduce the complexity of existence to the confines of the body itself. This is an important incision. Cutting into the manifold of existence, these "doctors of deviance" perform a conceptual surgery. They cut off the veins and arteries the body shares with the social. By these acts of carving and dissection, they isolate deviance, confine it. These same practices were used to determine the origins of diseases like AIDS, syphilis, gonorrhea, herpes. They worked. Why not use them on the addictions? The body, being complex enough, prevents medical experts from looking elsewhere. They have found their Mecca, and they are joined in their celebration by the majority of society. The rumors of the medical model have come true. The deviant, the sick, the insane, the criminal, our social calamities, all find their origins in the body. Somewhere, hidden deep within the body, is the defect. The goal of the medical model: find it!

Does Gambling Fit within the Medical Model? Is It a Disease?

Differences aside, common to the major theoretical camps in the field of gambling studies—from neuro to cognitive psychology—is the belief that excessive gambling is within the theoretical and clinical jurisdiction of the medical model, and is a disease, a mental illness. It is only a matter of transferring the tools, techniques and theoretical devices of the medical model onto the problems of gambling. In the process, surely new ways of defining, understanding and treating gambling will emerge. Indeed they did. Historical evidence is found by listing a few of the more recent publications in the field of gambling studies: 1) "Pathological Gambling and Platelet MAO Activity: A Psychobiological Study" (Blanco, Orensanz-Munoz, Blanco-Jerez and Saiz-Ruiz, 1996), 2) "Low Platelet Monoamine Oxidase Activity in Pathological Gambling" (Carrasco, Saiz-Ruiz, Hollander and Cesar 1994), 3) "Treatment of Pathological Gambling with Carbamazepine" (Haller and Hinterhuber 1994), 4) "Treatment of Pathological Gambling with Clomipramine" (Hollander, Frenkel, Decaria, Trungold, et. al. 1992), 5) "Serotonin and Gambling Dependence" (Moreno, Saiz-Ruiz, Lopez-Ibor 1991), 6) "Plasma Cortisol and Depression in Pathological Gamblers" (Ramirez, McCormick, and Lowy 1988), 7) "CSF GABA and Neuropeptides in Pathological Gamblers and Normal Controls" (Roy, DeJong, Ferraro, Adinoff, et. al. 1989) and others (e.g., Griffith 1989; Roy 1991; Roy, Picker, Gold, Barbaccia, et al. 1989; Roy, Adinoff, Roehrich, Lamparski et. al. 1989; Roy, Berrettine, Adinoff, and Linnoila 1990).

Further evidence for the medical model's dominance in the field comes from a review of the past thirteen years of articles published in *The Journal of Gambling Studies*. To conduct this review, I read the titles, and if ambiguous, the abstracts, to determine if the medical model was used as the basis for the study. (For my definition of the medical model I used Conrad and Schneider 1980, p. 35.) Of the 204 articles I looked at, 76 percent of them (N = 155) fit Conrad and Schneider's definition of the medical model. Of these 155 articles, 56 percent (N = 85) focused on the symptoms and etiology of pathological gambling (e.g., depression levels in pathological gamblers); 13 percent (N = 22) focused on the psychological, neuro-cognitive and physiological factors that influence the activity of gambling itself (e.g., psychobiological correlates of dependent slot machine gambling in adults), and 31 percent (N = 48) focused on the topic of treatment (e.g., assessment, diagnosis and treatment procedures for pathological gamblers). And what about the remaining articles that did not adhere to the medical model? Of the total number of articles (N = 204), 7 percent (N = 15) focused on demographic and epidemiological information (e.g., How many adolescents gamble in the United States?); 8 percent (N = 17) focused on policy and political issues (e.g., Should gambling be legalized?); 3 percent (N = 7) focused on the economic and social consequences of excessive gambling; and 5 percent (N = 10) focused on sociological concerns (e.g., gambling as a form of social play). As this review suggests, despite variance, the scientific and clinical literature situates pathological gambling within the domain of the medical. Researchers situate pathological gambling this way because of its DSM diagnosis.

Defining Excessive Gambling as a Medical Problem

Experts within the medical model generally define excessive gambling according to DSM diagnostic nomenclature. The first complete nomenclature came with the 1980 publication of the DSM-III. The DSM-III criteria are as follows:

DSM-III Diagnostic Criteria for Pathological Gambling

A. The individual is chronically and progressively unable to resist impulses to gamble.

B. Gambling compromises, disrupts, or damages family, personal, and vocational pursuits, as indicated by at least three of the following:

(1) arrest for forgery, fraud, embezzlement, or income tax evasion due to attempts to obtain money for gambling

(2) default or debts or other financial responsibilities

(3) disrupted family or spouse relationship due to gambling

(4) borrowing of money from illegal sources (loan sharks)

(5) inability to account for loss of money or to produce evidence of winning money, if this is claimed

(6) loss of work due to absenteeism in order to pursue gambling activity

(7) necessity for another person to provide money to relieve a desperate financial situation

C. The gambling is not due to Antisocial Personality Disorder.

(American Psychiatric Association, DSM-III 1980).

According to criteria A and B of the DSM-III, pathological gambling is a mental illness which leads to a series of negative consequences. The consequences inflict the damage. The consequences (e.g., increased spending, debt, family disruption, marital troubles, problems at work, increased potential to commit a crime) are the cause of the problem; not gambling itself. If these consequences total three or more, then a diagnosis of pathological gambling is given. It is also important that the individual's gambling is not the result of an anti-social personality disorder. Anti-social individuals lie, cheat, steal, con, gamble and suffer from a failure to learn from the consequences of their behavior. Even though these are the same problems found in pathological gamblers, the difference—according to the DSM-III—is that anti-social personality disorder emerges from a personality defect, whereas pathological gambling is the result of a disorder of impulse control. If there is no comorbid anti-social personality disorder, then the diagnosis is given.

While the DSM-III diagnosis of pathological gambling was the first step toward defining pathological gambling, it was improved for the 1987 publication of the DSM-III-R. The diagnosis of pathological gambling in the DSM-III-R is as follows:

DSM-III-R Diagnostic Criteria for Pathological Gambling

Maladaptive gambling behavior, as indicated by at least four of the following:

(1) frequent preoccupation with gambling or with obtaining money to gamble

(2) frequent gambling of larger amounts of money or over a longer period of time than intended

(3) a need to increase the size or frequency of bets to achieve the desired excitement

(4) restlessness or irritability if unable to gamble

(5) repeated loss of money by gambling and returning another day to win back losses ("chasing")

(6) repeated efforts to reduce or stop gambling

(7) frequent gambling when expected to meet social or occupational obligations

(8) sacrifice of some important social, occupational, or recreational activity in order to gamble

(9) continuation of gambling despite inability to pay mounting debts, or despite other significant social, occupational, or legal problems that the person knows to be exacerbated by gambling. (American Psychiatric Association, DSM-III-R 1987)

As you can see, the definition of pathological gambling in the DSM-III-R is radically different from the DSM-III. There were a number of reasons for this change. One reason was the criminal justice literature. While the DSM-III was a major breakthrough in the medical understanding and treatment of pathological gambling, it quickly came under criticism within the criminal justice literature because the diagnosis was too often misused as an insanity defense (e.g., Cunnien 1985; Rachlin, Halpern, and Portnow 1986; Rubin 1982). The primary basis for gambling misuse as an insanity defense was the phrase: " [pathological gamblers are] chronically and progressively unable to resist impulses to gamble" (DSM-III 1980, p. 291).

Rachlin, Halpern and Portnow (1986) were particularly concerned about this phrase because they felt the DSM-III was a clinical, and not a legal, document. Its purpose, as a nomenclature, was "to enable us to treat, study, and communicate about mental disorders" (p. 239). Its use in court should proceed with caution. They stated that the DSM-III "specifies that its use for such purposes as determination of criminal responsibility must be critically examined in the particular context" (p. 239). The loose handling of pathological gambling, based on the statement that pathological gamblers "are unable to resist the impulse to gamble" (DSM-III 1980, p. 291) obviously troubled them. They felt that the wording, while understood clinically, did not accurately reflect the legal definition of responsibility. They were therefore pleased that the revised edition of the DSM replaced "the foregoing phrase with the more proper statement 'failure to resist'" (1987, p. 239).

In addition to problems with the wording, another concern was that the diagnosis did not accurately portray pathological gambling as an addiction. In their article on the reconstruction of pathological gambling for the DSM-III-R, Lesieur and Rosenthal (1991) made explicit their intention to define pathological gambling as an *addiction.* In fact, they stated that their construction of the DSM-III-R criteria was "specifically modeled after those for psychoactive substance dependence in the DSM-III revision" (p. 8). Every one of the nine criteria, except "chasing losses," had "their counterpart in the diagnosis of alcohol, heroin, cocaine and other forms of drug dependence" (p. 8). And they were likewise clear that this change in orientation from a compulsion to an addiction would have "great implications for the study and treatment of pathological gambling" (p. 9).

Still, while the DSM-III-R diagnosis was considered an improvement over the DSM-III, clinicians continued, over the next several years, to voice their complaints to Lesieur and Rosenthal (Rosenthal, along with Lesieur, is another important name in the field of gambling studies) that further revision was still necessary. To counteract these problems Lesieur and Rosenthal did research to correct past errors and respond to complaints. Their new version of pathological gambling came out in the 1994 publication of the DSM-IV. This time the changes were less radical. The primary concern was, again, the need to make gambling more like an addiction. The other problem was the lack of distinction between criterion seven, eight and nine of the DSM-III-R. To handle these concerns, Lesieur and Rosenthal (1991) constructed a questionnaire based on the old DSM-III and DSM-III-R criteria for pathological gambling, to which they added a number of additional questions based on suggestions made by several top clinicians in the field. They then gave the questionnaire to "222 (164 males and 57 female) pathological gamblers as well as 104 (80 males and

24 female) substance abusing controls (controls were 'social gamblers,' none gambled rarely or never)" (p. 9). Lesieur and Rosenthal then took the results from the questionnaire and performed an "item analysis" to "determine which items discriminated between self-described 'compulsive gambler' and controls" (p. 9). Based on their research they constructed the following diagnostic criteria:

DSM-IV Diagnostic Criteria for Pathological Gambling

A. Persistent and recurrent maladaptive gambling behavior as indicated by five (or more) of the following:

(1) is preoccupied with gambling (e.g., preoccupied with reliving past gambling experiences, handicapping or planning the next venture, or thinking of ways to get money with which to gamble)

(2) needs to gamble with increasing amounts of money in order to achieve the desired excitement.

(3) has repeated unsuccessful efforts to control, cut back, or stop gambling

(4) is restless or irritable when attempting to cut down or stop gambling

(5) gambles as a way of escaping from problems or of relieving a dysphoric mood (e.g., feelings of helplessness, guilt, anxiety, depression)

(6) after losing money gambling, often returns another day to get even ("chasing" one's losses)

(7) lies to family members, therapist, or others to conceal the extent of involvement with gambling

(8) has committed illegal acts such as forgery, fraud, theft, or embezzlement to finance gambling

(9) has jeopardized or lost a significant relationship, job, or educational or career opportunity because of gambling

(10) relies on others to provide money to relieve a desperate financial situation caused by gambling

B. The gambling behavior is not better accounted for by a Manic Episode. (American Psychiatric Association, DSM-IV 1994)

The DSM-IV is the most current form of diagnostic criteria used in the treatment of pathological gambling. From the perspective of the current study, there are a number of problems with this diagnostic criteria which lead to the perpetuation of the medical model.

What Makes Pathological Gambling a Medical Problem?

The interesting thing about pathological gambling is that, unlike other addictions, it does not involve the ingestion, and consequently dependence upon, an external substance, such as cocaine, heroin or alcohol. It is a behavior. Because it is a behavior and does not meet the standard definition of addiction, it is catalogued in the DSM-IV (American Psychiatric Association 1994) as an impulse control disorder.

If, according to the DSM-IV, gambling does not meet the standards of an addiction and is a behavior, how does it become problematic? As the above ten symptoms found in the DSM-IV diagnosis illustrate, the problems of pathological gambling have to do with the relationship individuals have with the activity of gambling itself. If and when people become "addicted" to—that is, they significantly increase their involvement with—gambling, they often encounter a series of unintended consequences that are a direct result of the "losing phase" of gambling (Rosecrance 1985b). Once gamblers begin to lose money (or have a big win) they begin to gamble more and more to make up the loss (or repeat the first big win). Of course they hardly ever make up the money immediately, and so they become involved in a chase, a chase to win back their losses (Lesieur 1977). It is during the chase that people get into trouble. If they continue to gamble too much they may lose a great deal of income. They may begin to lie to their family, become depressed, feel anxious or suicidal, steal from their friends and employers, fail to show up for work, lose interest in the rest of their lives and loved ones, become obsessed with winning itself, turn to a life of crime, and so on. Surprisingly enough, often the losing phase is short-term and individuals somehow manage to cover up their mistakes, perhaps by another "big win" or a "bail out" from family and friends. Over time, though, these individuals repeat the behavior enough so that others begin to catch on. Soon they have lost too much money or have ruined too many relationships, or actually get caught stealing and go to jail, or even seek medical or mental health treatment for the emotional and physical consequences of their actions, and so their gambling comes to an end, at least for the moment. It is at these points that individuals often receive the diagnosis of pathological gambling, and so their problems become medicalized.

Given the typical pattern of most individuals diagnosed with pathological gambling, it appears that the problem is not the gambling itself but the individual's involvement in the chase. The real question to answer, therefore, is why do people become addicted to the chase? The answer is that people become addicted to the "chase" for reasons other than the gambling itself. Restated, it is not because of gambling itself, but for reasons other than it, that some people are more likely than others to become involved in the chase of pathological gambling. Once the individual is involved in the chase these "other" factors become wrapped up in the gambling making it difficult to determine just what is causing what. It is this confusion between what is causing what that makes the medical model plausible. The medical model gives the impression that the problems of pathological gambling are a result of the gambling itself, when, in fact, the problems were there before the chase became a problem. If we were to tease out the relationship between these predisposing factors and the gambling itself, the limitations of the medical model would emerge.

To tease out the relationship between gambling and its predisposing factors we need to take a closer look at the symptoms comprising the DSM-IV. If you notice, all ten symptoms can be lumped into three general categories: those which describe the initial reasons for becoming involved in pathological gambling (symptom five), those which describe the chase itself (symptoms one, two, three, four and six) and those which describe its consequences (symptoms seven, eight, nine and ten). If we were to put these symptoms in order, we would get a story similar to the one above: For various reasons, which can range from problems with impulsivity to economic depression, certain individuals are more likely than others to use gambling as a way to escape—that is, avoid or cope with—the problems in their life. Once they gamble, they often become involved in the chase. Once in the chase, these individuals, for reasons other than the gambling itself, become addicted to the chase. They are hooked. The factors their pathological gambling becomes involved with range from attention deficit disorder, lack of ego integration and gender role strain to marital discord, dissatisfaction with life, and even genetics. As their involvement in the chase repeats itself, they also suffer a number of unintended consequences: depression, anxiety, job loss, bankruptcy, criminal prosecution, divorce, family discord, etc. It is the consequences of the chase that often invite the attention of the medical expert. Once noticed, these behaviors are interpreted from within the framework of the medical model. This is the process of becoming a pathological gambler.

So what does all of this mean for researchers in the field of gambling studies? If they wish to do medical research—and by that I mean research that "locates the sources of deviant behavior within the individual, postulating a physiological, constitutional, organic, or, occasionally, psychogenic agent or condition that is assumed to cause the behavioral deviance" (Conrad and Schneider 1980, p. 35)—they cannot ground their work in the chase itself. They have to focus on the predisposing factors which perpetuate the chase. Not in any of the medical theories currently existing is gambling defined as a disease unto itself. Each and every one of the theories—all of them—have to leave gambling to search for a foundation in other parts of the body. Some venture inward into the brain, beyond its neurotransmittors to the cortex, to the frontal lobe. There they find neuropsychological and structural deficits (e.g., Carlton and Manowitz 1992; Carroll and Huxley 1994). Onward still, some venture into the memory and its cognitive tangles. There they find repressed memories from childhood, neural fibers filled with restricted affect waiting to be released (e.g., Blaszczynski and Silove 1995; Rugle 1993). Others explore perceptual problems, behavioral reward systems, and difficulties with cognition and attention. There they find children in adult bodies unable to handle the stimuli and stressors of the chase (e.g., Carlton, Manowitz, McBride and Nora 1987; Rugle and Melamed 1993). Still others, unconvinced to stop at the level of chemistry or cognition, go further into the body. Raising the focus of the microscope to even higher levels of power, these individuals search the genetic codes of life hoping to find a connection, a flaw, an error on the double-helix (Comings, Rosenthal, Lesieur, Rugle, et al. 1996). These are the theoretico-empirical variants of the medical model. All of them, despite their differences, ground pathological gambling in one or another more "real" diseases of the brain or body to give pathological gambling its medical status. Let's review some examples.

Examples from the Literature

The field of gambling studies is a small field and has a short history. Most of the medical research got its start in the middle 1980s and became popular during the 1990s. Examples of the research include titles such as 1) "Pathological Gambling and Platelet MAO Activity: A Psychobiological Study" (Blanco, Orensanz-Munoz, Blanco-Jerez and Saiz-Ruiz 1996), 2) "Low Platelet Monoamine Oxidase Activity in Pathological Gambling" (Carrasco, Saiz-Ruiz, Hollander and Cesar 1994), 4) "Serotonin and Gambling Dependence" (Moreno, Saiz-Ruiz, Lopez-Ibor 1991), 5) "Plasma Cortisol and Depression in Pathological Gamblers" (Ramirez, McCormick, and Lowy 1988), and 6) "CSF GABA and Neuropeptides in Pathological Gamblers and Normal Controls" (Roy, DeJong, Ferraro, Adinoff, et. al. 1989).

The primary strategy used in the research is as follows. First, some comorbid medical condition is found which is believed to be related to pathological gambling. For example, a clinician reports problems with impulsivity in his or her treatment population. The research is then conducted by determining the prevalence of the comorbid condition in relation to a control group or another treatment population, such as people with alcoholism or drug dependence. If the results are statistically significant, a new comorbid medical predisposition is found, which allows pathological gambling to be replaced by the comorbid condition as the focus of study. Medical researchers then argue with one another about which predisposing comorbid factor accounts for the greatest percentage of variance.

Of the various medical comorbid conditions researched, problems with attention deficit, impulsivity, arousal, sensation seeking, and cognitive appraisal are the most studied. Researchers working in this area establish their laboratory at the threshold points where neurological and perceptual hardware meet, intersect with, are affected by, cognition and emotion. The gambling object of investigation created is the neurotransmitter, the neurological tangle, the biochemical imbalance, the cognitive impairment. The neuropsychological models are highly interactive. They see the gambling individual as a weave of interconnecting mental, emotional, and physical systems which, while never complete, form the larger working system known as the gambling individual (e.g., Carroll and Huxley 1994). This larger working system, through its interactions with the environment, has certain vulnerabilities which, if pushed, can break down or cause problems (e.g., Black, Goldstein, Noyes, and Blume 1994; Carlton and Manowitz 1992; Castellani and Rugle 1995; Cocco, Sharpe, and Blaszczynski 1995; Goldstein and Carlton 1988; McCormick 1988; Roy, Berrettine, Adinoff, Linnoila 1990; Rugle 1993; Rugle and Melamed 1993; Sharpe, Tarrier, Schotte and Spence 1995; Sharpe and Nicholas 1995).

One of the better theoretical models illustrating how pathological gambling is grounded in neuropsychology comes from the work of Loreen Rugle. She has published two important articles in this area: "Neuropsychological Assessment of Attention Problems in Pathological Gamblers" (Rugle and Melamed 1993), and "Initial Thoughts on Viewing Pathological Gambling from a Physiological and Intrapsychic Structural Perspective" (Rugle 1993). Because she is a leader in the field, her work is a standard by which the field is defined.

Rugle (1993) defines her theoretical framework as structural because it is based on two important premises: "1) deficits in key physiological and intrapsychic structures are risk factors for pathological gambling as well as other addictive disorders, and 2) such structural deficits contribute to addictive individuals' difficulties in organizing their experience in effectively adaptive ways" (p. 4). Using this framework, Rugle explains that pathological gamblers are at risk for addiction because they lack the cognitive and perceptual structures needed to understand and cope with their emotional and intrapsychic problems, as well as deal with the physical and social environments in which they live. These problematic internal structures, however, are not the result of pathological gambling; they are its cause. As intrapsychic imbalances interact with cognitive distortions and difficulties with impulsivity and attention, certain individuals become involved in the chase of gambling and find themselves unable to control their behavior long enough to stop their gambling. They become engaged in a cycle of abuse that results in increasing levels of gambling dependence. As these problems progress, the cycle becomes harder and harder to break because dysfunctions in so many different inter-dependent systems feed off one another. The end result is the pathological gambling condition.

Given the complexity of comorbid associations found at the neuropsychological and intrapsychic level, most researchers do not engage in the level of sophistication suggested by Rugle's work. Instead they strive for parsimony (ergo psychological reductionism) by choosing one or two variables most likely to explain the greatest amount of variance. The variables most often chosen are impulsivity and attention deficit disorder (see Lesieur and Rosenthal 1991).

For example, in their article "Attention Deficit Disorder and Pathological Gambling," Carlton, Manowitz, Mcbride and Nora (1987) examined pathological gamblers to determine if they showed "high levels of ADD-related behavior during childhood" (p. 487). They examined childhood ADD levels because previous research had suggested that "subtle EEG deficits found in recovered pathological gamblers parallel those found in children with attention deficit disorder (ADD)" (p. 487). To complete their study, Carlton et al. compared 14 pathological gamblers to 16 controls on issues related to childhood ADD and found that the self reports "indicated a strong correlation between pathological gambling and childhood behaviors related to attention deficit disorder" (p. 487). As in Rugle's theoretical model, Carlton et al. did not study pathological gambling. They studied the prevalence levels of childhood ADD. Their focus was on a comorbid—or what we could call a pre-comorbid—condition that may have been the primary cause of their subjects' adult onset of pathological gambling.

Another example comes from Specker, Carlson, Christenson and Marcottte's (1995) article, "Impulse Control Disorders and Attention Deficit Disorder in Pathological Gamblers." In their article, ADD and impulsivity were specifically referred to as comorbid problems. They stated: "Little systematic research has been done on the psychiatric comorbidity of pathological gambling, an impulse control disorder" (p. 175). Their study examined 40 pathological gamblers in comparison to 64 controls to see if there was a significant difference in levels of attention deficit and impulsive control. Their conclusions were the same as Rugle (1993) and Carlton et al. (1987). Although the differences weren't significant, pathological gamblers were higher in ADD and impulse control disorder than the controls. Again, pathological gambling, as its own problem, was not studied. The focus was on the prevalence of two other, more real, medical disorders—impulsivity and ADD—which, again, according to them, may be the primary cause of pathological gambling.

Research in the psychophysiology of pathological gambling reveals the same discursive strategies. Examples of recent studies include 1) "Physiological Determinants Of Pathological Gambling" by Carlton and Goldstein (1987) and 2) "Low Platelet Monoamine Oxidase Activity in Pathological Gambling" by Carrasco, Saiz-Ruiz, Hollander, and Cesar (1994). In their study on monoamine oxidase (MAO) activity in pathological gamblers, Carrasco and colleagues (1994) argued that while studies had been done on the intrapsychic aspects of pathological gambling, "little is known about its biological correlates" (p.119). They, therefore, studied "platelet MAO activity in pathological gamblers in an attempt to find a biological correlate for the characteristic impulsivity of the disorder" (p. 119). Again, this study was an issue of prevalence. Carrasco and colleagues wanted to know what type of MAO activity occurred in individuals diagnosed with pathological gambling in comparison to controls. Once the prevalence was found statistically significant, the association between the two heterogeneous factors (MAO activity and pathological gambling) was made: a causal direction was assumed and inferred, running from the predisposing comorbid condition to pathological gambling itself—not the other way around.

Even in the medical research that studies the act of gambling itself the focus is on problems elsewhere. These problems include cognitive distortions ("Cognitive, Dispositional, and Psychobiological Correlates of Dependent Slot Machine Gambling in Young People," Douglas and Huxley 1994), perceptual biases ("Erroneous Perceptions and Arousal Among Regular and Occasional Video Poker Players," by Cloulombe, Ladouceur, Desharnais, and Jobin 1992), and problems with arousal states and compulsive behavior ("Differences in Preferred Level of Arousal in Two Sub-Groups of Problem Gamblers: A Preliminary Report," by Cocco, Sharpe, and Blaszczynski 1995). For example, in Kroeber's (1992) study of the differences between pathological gamblers who play roulette and electronic machines, he focused on the constellation of complex psycho-social factors that statistically distinguished the two groups. Those who played the electronic games, such as video poker, started gambling around the age of nineteen, while roulette gamblers started much later, around twenty-eight. Electronic gamblers were also more often from the lower class and displayed, on average, a higher percentage of depressive and reactive disorders, whereas roulette gamblers "showed signs of personality disorders, especially narcissistic and cyclothymic patterns, significantly more often" (p. 79). And so, similar to the examples above, Kroeber's study did not research gambling itself; it examined the factors which he believed responsible for its activity. The causal arrows run from the social and the physiological and perceptual to the behavior of gambling, not the other way around.

And finally, there is the genetic research, the most important research of all. Consistent with the above studies, researchers in this area do not ground their work in the disorder of pathological gambling itself. Like everyone else, they focus on the prevalence of their specified pre-comorbid condition, the gene.

To date, three articles have been written on the genetics of pathological gambling: two are by David Comings and colleagues (1996, 1997) and the third is by a research group in Spain, Perez de Castro, Ibanez ,Torres, et al. (1997). Differences between the three articles aside, the same argument is made as above: a comorbid precondition, in this case genetics, is one of the primary reasons why pathological gambling exists. The gene itself, be it located at the D1, D2, or D4 receptor cite, doesn't matter. What matters is that pathological gamblers have significantly higher levels of the gene than their comparison group, be they a control or treatment sample. The article best illustrative of this area of research is Comings et al. 1996 article, titled "A Study of the Dopamine Receptor Gene in Pathological Gambling." In the second paragraph they put forth their hypothesis: "Since the accumulated findings to date suggest that genetic variants at the DRD2 locus may play a role in the genetic susceptibility to addictive-compulsive behaviors, we have sought to determine if a similar relationship might be present with pathological gambling. A variant of the dopamine D3 receptor gene was also examined" (1996, p. 224).

In the words of Comings and his colleagues, the focus of their article was to determine if there is an association between the DRD2 receptor site and pathological gambling. This defect, they explained, has been found in a variety of other addictive populations, including alcoholics, smokers and drug addicts. It has also been found in people with Tourette syndrome, hyperactivity, attention deficit disorder, conduct disorder, and post-traumatic stress disorder. They hoped to find it in pathological gamblers as well. They did: "The results showed a significant increase in both the prevalence of the D_2A1 allele in 171 pathological gamblers (50.9%) compared to 714 non-Hispanic Caucasian controls (25.9%). The frequency of the D_2A1 allele was also significantly increased" (1996, p. 229). In fact, the more prevalent the genetic variant was, the greater the level of gambling severity reported. This suggested that there are people who are vulnerable to certain activities such as gambling because they are genetically predisposed to problems with impulse control, addiction, compulsion, and attention. They are poor planners and have difficulty delaying gratification or thinking before acting. This research therefore supported "a role for genetic defects in the dopaminergic reward pathways and the DRD2 gene in pathological gambling and addictive behaviors in general" (Comings et al., 1996, p. 232).

But, according to the research of Comings and his colleagues, the DRD2 gene is not directly related to gambling. People with a DRD2 receptor problem could just as easily get involved in a variety of other impulsive and repetitive behaviors. Their impulsivity could interfere with business decisions, financial engagements and so on. Why, then, are these people choosing to gamble so much? They gamble for a whole host of different reasons. One of the reasons happens to be problems with impulsivity and ADD, which can be related to genetic dysfunction. At this time, then, all that can be reported is that people who have a DRD2 defect are likely to have problems with impulsivity, attention deficit disorder and compulsive behavior and are, therefore, at risk for the excesses and problems of pathological gambling. The genetic explanation of gambling is an indirect explanation and should only be addressed in relation to other factors such as the psychological, sociological, economic, political and cultural.

Why Medical Researchers Make the Arguments They Do

So why do these researchers make the arguments they do? There are many reasons. A good percentage of the reasons are institutional, organizational, political, economic, personal, and professional, but these are issues for the rest of the book. What I am most concerned about in this chapter is the research itself: I want to know what linguistic slight of hand allows these researchers to assume that they've made pathological gambling into a medical object of investigation.

The answer has to do with the DSM diagnosis of pathological gambling itself and its effect on the nature of medical inquiry. The diagnosis of pathological gambling is a list of symptoms only. Once an individual is diagnosed, her complex etiology is forgotten. The problem is de-contextualized. The fact that pathological gambling, as a behavior, is multipley determined doesn't matter, and the fact that pathological gambling is a heterogeneous category is of no concern. Why one person gets involved in the "chase" versus another is not an issue; that is, until it comes time to do research. Then, all of a sudden, etiology becomes everything because without it pathological gambling cannot be studied medically. Thus, starting with their decontextualized sample of patients—who have little in common with one another other than a diagnosis—researchers try to find the one key factor they believe will re-contextualize their otherwise heterogeneous sample. The variable chosen may be impulsivity or ADD. It doesn't matter. All that matters is that the variable explain a significant percentage of the variance. As soon as the variable is found, the larger spectrum of relevant factors is forgotten and replaced by a new, albeit radically limited, etiological context which is grounded in the medical model alone. Medical reductionism is secured.

Having accomplished their goal of reductionism, it becomes easy for medical researchers, in the name of parsimony, to wrestle with one another to assert their variable as more important than the others. Given this field of competition, research quickly becomes a game between scientists. In fact, over the past fifteen years it has been through the discursive play of the above researchers that pathological gambling has emerged as a medical object of investigation. Because of their search for those one or two variables that will explain pathological gambling, they have not only ignored each other, they have also ignored the larger and smaller social contexts in which the "chase" takes place. And they have ignored the complex, etiologically nuanced, highly contextualized lives of their patients. As a result, they have understood very little about the problem they believe themselves to be studying.

Chapter 4

THE DEFENSE'S ARGUMENT

Now that we have a basic understanding of the medical model of pathological gambling itself, it's time to return to the argument put forth by Torniero's defense to better understand the political context within which the medical research has been situated.

Torniero's defense attorneys, Keefe and Keefe, had two basic goals. They wanted to convince the judge that "1. Pathological gambling is a mental disease or defect within the meaning of the ALI rules; [and] 2. A pathological gambler is unable to resist impulses to gambling and may, therefore, lack substantial capacity to refrain from engaging in criminal activity such as interstate transportation of stolen goods and similar offenses" (United States of America v. John Torniero, No. 83–1459, Brief for the Appellant, p. 15).

To accomplish their task, Keefe and Keefe brought in the leading authorities on pathological gambling. They had the best. Their list included Robert Custer, M.D., Julian Taber, Ph.D., Ernest Prelinger, Ph.D. (a clinical psychologist at Yale University), Monsignor Joseph A. Dunne (president of the National Council of Compulsive Gambling) and Patricia Nere, M.S.W., (Director of the Connecticut Statewide Treatment Program for Compulsive Gambling in Bridgeport). During the 1980s and 1990s, the above intellectuals were primary proponents of the medical model of pathological gambling, particularly Robert Custer, who started the Brecksville Gambling Treatment Program in 1972, and Monsignor Dunne, who started the National Council on Problem Gambling.

In addition to the above list of stars, Keefe brought in Dr. Robert Matefy, a clinical psychologist at the University of Bridgeport in Connecticut. At the time of the trial, Matefy was in private practice and had written an article (1983) for the National Council on Problem Gambling, titled "Is Compulsive Gambling Treatable?" During the five years prior to the court case, Matefy devoted a considerable amount of his practice to the treatment of pathological gamblers and their families. We join the court trial about a quarter of the way through Matefy's testimony. Keefe is doing the questioning:

BY MR. KEEFE:

Q Dr. Matefy, we will get back to your diagnosing procedure in a moment, but before we do, sir, you are familiar with the American Law Institute standards for legal insanity, is that correct?

A I am. . . .

Q And, sir, in your opinion, based on your experience with pathological gamblers, sir, is pathological gambling a mental disease or defect?

A Yes.

Q And which is it, disease or defect; or in your opinion does it make any difference?

A I think they are used interchangeably.

Q And in some instances, sir, do you have an opinion as to whether a person who suffers from the disease of pathological gambling is substantially incapable of conforming his conduct to the requirements of law?

A During certain stages of the disorder he is unable to conform. . . .

Q And how disturbed are pathological gamblers, how serious a mental illness or mental disease is that?

A I see the pathological gambler potentially as being a very severe disorder. In its progression at its lowest point it is very severe.

Q And what do you mean by that?

A What I'm trying to do is distinguish between—you know, it's a progressive disorder, of course. When it has progressed to the point of desperation, it is among the most severe disorders I know of. . . . (United States vs. John J. Torniero, 1983 Criminal 82–1106, pp. 328–330)

In the above initial sets of questions, Keefe is trying to convince the judge that pathological gambling is as severe as, or potentially even more severe than, other mental diseases. So far he has gotten Matefy to agree with him. Now, his goal is to show just how severe the gambling is.

BY MR. KEEFE:

Q And what other symptoms do pathological gamblers suffer?

A Depression, deep depression. As a matter of fact, oftentimes the gambling is an attempt to escape from the depression.

A great deal of self-reproach and remorse for the harm they've done to others—one of the distinctions between a pathological gambler, by the way, and other kinds of gamblers that are not pathological gamblers.

They often come from homes in early childhood that are unstable, emotionally deprived. That seems to be a major factor.

There is gambling reinforced in the family. It's another sign I look for. Usually there's a role model of a gambler.

One person said to me, he said, "I don't have any role models, my mother and father never gambled in their lives." Then it turned out, though, that his mother was at the bingo table seven nights a week, and that's where he would meet her.

Very importantly, their socially-responsible behavior typically is confined to and a direct result of their desperate stage where they require funds to continue their gambling.

> Up to that point, for the most part, I find that they tend not to be irresponsible; on the contrary, as a matter of fact, they tend to be very responsible individuals. Usually the crimes that they commit to support their gambling habits are non-violent in nature. Often there is at least a superficial intent to pay back the child's piggy bank, the wife's vacation funds, and so on. (United States vs. John J. Torniero, 1983 Criminal 82–1106, pp. 330–331)

After Matefy left the witness stand, Keefe brought in other witnesses to likewise testify about the severity of pathological gambling. All of them, like Matefy, made the same argument: gambling is a severe and destructive disease and is as pathological as other mental illnesses. Monsignor Dunne, the president of the National Council, told a story about a friend of his who was a compulsive gambler: "His wife says to him, 'Julie, when you were gambling what did I mean to you?' He is dying of cancer. . . . He looked at her and said, 'When I was gambling you were not even a stick of furniture.' That's the compulsive gambler. Totally unrelated to reality."[1]

Keefe's expert witnesses, including Dunne and Matefy, also agreed that, in addition to being a serious mental illness, in the final stages of pathological gambling, which they called the desperation phase, gamblers are at their worst. Patricia Nere, Director of the Connecticut Statewide Treatment Program for Compulsive Gamblers explained that: "By this point in time they have given up everything, practically, to continue to gamble. Nothing means anything in their life at all. Their families don't, their children don't. I've heard gamblers say they don't even know what season it is.[2] Custer was equally adamant: "I think in the desperation phase they of course are starting the day off thinking of gambling only. They are very restless, uncommunicative, they have little direction as to where they are going. They don't communicate well at all with people around them. And if they do, it is very fragmented. Nobody can quite understand what they are saying."[3]

"Nothing around them is real anymore," said Nere. "They engage in a great amount of magical thinking and think they can control everything. They are very turned on by the action and cannot stop and without the action life has no meaning for them."[4] Julian Taber went into greater depth about the desperation phase. "To describe his psychological functioning, he is often in a panic state, he is not thinking clearly in terms of his alternatives. As Dr. Custer stated, he sees gambling as the solution to the problems rather than the cause of the problems. Frequently he is troubled by feelings of disassociation. These are feelings of not being really part of yourself. Gamblers frequently describe to me a feeling of being separate from the scene, of standing and looking on. Frequently they are alienated, they have no one they can talk to, no one they can trust."[5]

Keefe and Keefe were beginning to build a strong case with these testimonies. Between the 21st and 29th of June 1983, the judge heard from the defense's witnesses.

Building on these testimonies, Custer continued to go deeper into the problems that emerge during the desperation phase: "Their judgement on any matter is seriously impaired. They are erratic even in driving an automobile. People will avoid riding with them. They are unconcerned about eating. They are unconcerned about sleep, they are unconcerned about sex, they show no affection whatsoever, they seem to be in a world of their own and in a tremendous amount of personal torment, there seems to be a painful agonizing thing for them, and they will describe that."[6] Taber added to Custer by explaining what happens to work, "Vocationally they've lost probably most jobs or are just hanging on, although in the pathological gambler you see a loyalty to the trade or the profession they follow. They've often lost it because of gambling."[7] Taber also mentioned the family: "The family is usually chaotic, and frequently they've lost their wives and their children, and they have no place to live. Many of our gamblers report living in cars, living in friends' homes, wherever they can find a place."[8]

To increase the court's understanding of pathological gambling's severity, Keefe asked some of his witnesses to compare it to other major mental disorders that would normally fit within the domain of the insanity defense. They were willing and able.

Keefe had something going. He knew that if he could get the judge to see these similarities, the first part of his argument would be secure. "[A] large number of our outpatients are diagnosable as severely depressed," testified Taber. "About 30% have manic or hypomanic tendencies. They are, in fact, psychotic when we see them in the criminal stage."[9] Taber explained that because the gambler is so sick, gambling is an "extremely dehumanizing experience." "[T]hey are alienated and distrustful, even paranoid about family and loved ones. They suffer from considerable incorrect or delusional thinking along with the idea that they can beat the odds, that they can win it back—when, in fact, the money no longer exists in reality. And it's very hard for us to convince them that their thinking is distorted and incorrect and delusional."[10]

Keefe's argument was getting stronger. He asked Custer if pathological gamblers can become psychotic. Custer said "yes." Custer stated: "For some reason or other, pathological gambling has not ever been considered a serious disorder, and I think it is an exceptionally serious disorder. I think that it has all of the psychotic proportions, in some of them, not in all of them. But it is a mind that is totally out of control. And yet we think of them as dumb, naive, poor bettors, or something of that nature. But they're laughed at generally. But they're terribly sick people."[11]

Getting the needed backing from Custer, Keefe took his argument one step further. He asked Dr. Katz if pathological gambling was comparable to schizophrenia. Katz responded, "Well, Karl Menninger once said that if one of his children would have to develop schizophrenic disorder or a psychopathic disorder—one might put compulsive gambling under the old general rubric of psychopathic disorder—he said he would prefer his child suffer from schizophrenic illness because one might be able to help him or her, while it's much more difficult in these situations."[12] This is a powerful statement: pathological gambling is worse than full-blown schizophrenia! Keefe's witnesses were zealous to make their point.

Keefe, commenting on the testimony of Katz, stated later in his brief that, "The aforementioned testimony forcefully depicts the seriousness of the mental disease of pathological gambling and should [be] . . . more than sufficient for the court to determine that pathological gambling constitutes an allegation of a mental disease or defect for purposes of insanity. The testimony also meets the criteria required by the trial court in order for an insanity defense to be put before the jury in that it shows that at the point that the pathological gambler reaches the desperation phase, his mental state is 'such that the jury could not comprehend it.'"[13] Thus, argued Keefe, pathological gambling is severe enough and within the limits of the ALI test of insanity. Keefe's final witness, Dr. Prelinger, Chief Clinical Psychologist, at Yale University concurred with Keefe's conclusions: "So if the gambling disorder reaches a degree of severity in which, for instance, a person's reality testing is seriously impaired, . . . then I think the disorder has reached the proportion of serious mental disease and can qualify for the ALI formula."[14]

Having made his case about the severity of pathological gambling and its similarities to clinical depression, anxiety and psychosis, Keefe next tried to establish a causal link between pathological gambling and criminal behavior. Keefe's argument was along the following lines. First of all, he makes it clear that according to DSM-III criteria, "The overriding element of pathological gambling is characterized by the inability of the pathological gambler to control his conduct with respect to gambling."[15] Because the gambler lacks control over her behavior, if her gambling gets in the way of other decisions and behaviors, such as picking the kids up from school or coming home at night, these aspects of the gambler's life fall prey to the gambler's insanity and suffer as well. What adds to the insane behavior of the gambler is their constant need for money. They gamble so hard they are always running out of money. To compensate, they begin to do whatever is necessary to get money: lie, cheat, steal, con and so on. Putting this all together, because pathological gamblers, in their desperation phase, are as insane as a psychotic person, and because they have no control over their impulses and are in desperate need of money, it makes perfect sense that they could easily engage in criminal behavior, such as stealing, without understanding what they are doing. They do not steal because they are criminals. They steal because they are insane. The second half of the expert testimony was conducted to validate Keefe's argument. We again return to the testimony of Matefy:

BY MR. KEEFE:

Q [Mr. Matefy,] do some pathological gamblers commit crimes?"

A Yes.

Q Are the crimes they commit, based on your experience, to support their habit?

A Yes, and that's a very important qualifier to differentiate from, let's say, the anti-social personality.

One of the major things I look for in a differential diagnosis is that any criminal behavior is the direct result of the gambling, the uncontrollable urge to gamble, and is an attempt to support that gambling habit.

Q And in your opinion, sir, are pathological gamblers substantially incapable of resisting activity to get money to support their habit, activities such as embezzlement or fraud?

A In my experience in the five years I found to my astonishment that they are incapable of conforming.

Q Are the crimes that pathological gamblers commit to support their habit in your experience essentially of a non-violent nature?

A Yes.

Q And are they so-called white collar crimes that we have characterized?

A One way of putting it, yes. (United States vs. John J. Torniero, 1983 Criminal 82–1106, pp. 337–338)

Again, to strengthen the basic argument made by Matefy, Keefe turned to other witnesses. Regarding the inability of the pathological gambler to control her behavior, Monsignor Dunne testified:

> They are completely out of control of gambling and/or its aspects. Their every waking moment is taken up in calculating bets and raising money not only to pay debts, but also to be in action that day. This is essential to a compulsive gambler's life, to be in action. This is the only way he can deal or she can deal with the pain, the terrible pain, the guilt, the conflicts, the resentment, the remorse that this individual is left afflicting everyone around him. The only way they can find peace [is] to have gambling activity going on in their life. And I can give you thousands and thousands of examples of this phenomenon around the country.[16]

Patricia Nere said the same thing, "We find that with compulsive gamblers, they have been unable throughout their life to internalize anything, any external controls."[17] So did Custer, "I feel at that time they've lost control. Their judgement is so impaired and all that is on their mind is to gamble. And it interferes with every other aspect of their lives."[18] Taber expanded, "In the terminal stages the impulse is with him probably 24 hours a day; so, of course, he is not able to resist the impulse."[19] That's why," argued Nere, "Gamblers Anonymous and things like that are very important to help them continue to abstain or to control their impulses, because they have no internal control over their impulses at all."[20]

Having these strong statements from the witnesses out before the court, Keefe moved to the next step in his argument stating that because of the uncontrolled nature of the pathological gambler, "[i]t does not require a big leap in reasoning to conclude that being unable to resist impulses to gamble would require constant sums of money. Gambling is an appetite which must be fed with money. Therefore, it is apparent . . . that some gamblers may also lack substantial capacity to resist the opportunity to engage in criminal activity to support their uncontrollable desire to gamble."[21] Dunne supported Keefe's argument stating that once caught in the cycle of chasing her losses, the pathological gambler "will stoop to crime, will stoop to theft, embezzlement of funds; normally not violent crimes."[22] Custer agreed as well: "When they are in the desperation phase, they must gamble, they are driven to gamble, and they will do almost anything they can to obtain money in order to gamble. And with that, if they cannot get it legally or from an illegal source, such as a loan shark, then they may resort to committing a crime to get that money."[23] Taber made the final statement: "As a matter of fact, he may not even believe he is violating the law. One of the delusions may be that he is, in fact, borrowing money, he may believe that he knows a better use for the money than the proper owner. He is firmly convinced of this and intends to repay it—which is another one of his delusional systems."[24]

Given all of the testimony from the various experts in pathological gambling, Keefe believed he had made it clear that pathological gambling was proper grounds for the insanity defense and did lead very easily, in its more severe forms, to criminal behavior. He concluded his defense with the following statement: "Expert testimony regarding the Defendant's mental disorder, 'pathological gambling,' is properly admissible because pathological gambling is a mental disease or defect, as those terms are used in the ALI test of insanity, which renders the individual suffering from the disease substantially incapable of conforming his behavior to the requirements of law regulating interstate transportation of stolen goods."[25] With this statement the defense rested.

Chapter 5

IN-PATIENT TREATMENT

The witnesses called to testify on behalf of the defense during Torniero's trial played an important role in the history of pathological gambling, not only because of what they said during the trial but because of the larger social forces they each represented within the field of pathological gambling. The forces they represented totaled three: the field of gambling treatment, Gamblers Anonymous (GA), and the various state gambling councils located throughout the United States. Viewed together, what is interesting about these three forces is that, despite their differences, for the past three decades they've all remained true to the belief that pathological gambling is a diagnosable mental illness, an illness which affects roughly 3 percent of the general population. They've also all generally believed that research, clinical treatment, and education are the best approaches to solving the problem, and that the criminalization of this disorder provides no great benefit.

Given the similarities between these three positions, three questions immediately emerge. First of all, how and why did these three different forces come to the same basic conclusion that pathological gambling was a medical problem? Were the similarities in approach between these three forces a function of research and clinical investigation alone or were sociohistorical, political, institutional, professional, and economic factors involved as well? Second, how exactly did each of these forces use the medical model? Did they all use it in the same way? Did it mean the same thing to each of them? And third, what were the consequences of how they used it? What sort of impact did their acceptance of the medical model have on its creation, usage, and dissemination? To answer these questions, we start with the field of gambling treatment, then proceed to Gamblers Anonymous and the gambling councils.

The Medical Model of Gambling Treatment

So far in this study, I've offered two simultaneous, yet different, historical explanations for how the medical model was constructed. In the opening chapter, I argued that pathological gambling was constructed in response to the third wave of gambling legalization. From this perspective, the medical model made its mark on the history of gambling with the publication of the DSM-III. In chapter three, I changed gears. I offered a different explanation by decentering our study onto the field of gambling research itself. Starting with Conrad and Schneider's (1980) definition, I argued that the medical model emerged through the linguistic slight of hand researchers used to make pathological gambling into a medical object of investigation. In the present chapter, I offer yet another history. This time I argue that the medical model emerged out of Custer's establishment of the first in-patient gambling treatment center in the United States, the Brecksville Gambling Treatment Program.

To accomplish our task, we will proceed through several inter-connecting levels of socio-historical investigation. First, we will redefine the medical model according to Sheila Blume's (1987) article "Compulsive Gambling and the Medical Model." Blume's article provides an exhaustive explanation of what the medical model of gambling treatment is. Blume's definition is important because it shows that the medical model is not a monolithic structure; instead, it is a series of historically situated and inter-connected discursive strategies. Together, these strategies form the content and process of the medical model of gambling treatment. To further illustrate our point, we will review the concept of organizing practice (Castellani 1999). But, we don't stop there. As a concept, organizing practice also teaches us that the content and process of gambling treatment took place within a series of larger and smaller discursive practices which define its historical terms and conditions. Examples include the intentions and desires of Custer and members of Gamblers Anonymous, the changing health care system, and the opinions and practices of experts in the field of addiction treatment and research. Given this tension, we will end the chapter exploring how the content and process of the Brecksville Gambling Treatment Program was created as a function of the historical terms and conditions within which it emerged.

Redefining the Medical Model

What is the medical model of gambling treatment? Is it a discourse, a structure, a set of interactions, a way of thinking, a style of treatment? Or is it something entirely different? According to Sheila Blume, a well-known physician in the field of gambling studies and a colleague of Lesieur's (e.g., 1987, 1990, 1992), it is a combination of things, that's why she wrote "Compulsive Gambling and the Medical Model." She wanted to expand Conrad and Schneider's (1980) definition to include the numerous components most gambling treatment experts in the United States use.

According to Blume (1987), the medical model is comprised of the following important components. Each of these components, these practices, while part of the medical model itself, are their own strategy for approaching treatment. And, while also defined in terms of their shared inter-action with the others, each of these discursive strategies stand on their own. The first strategy defines "the individual" as the focal point of analysis and is grounded in individualism. The second looks for the origins of pathological gambling in the body while ignoring the process of gambling itself. These origins include the physiological, the neurological and the intra-psychic. The third situates pathological gambling within the theoretical and clinical jurisdiction of the medical model. And the fourth defines and treats it as a disease, a medical condition, a mental illness. The fifth transfers the tools, techniques and theoretical devices of the medical model onto the problems of gambling. The sixth hires professionals to do treatment, not just physicians, but psychiatric nurses, clinical psychologists, social workers, and certified addiction specialists as well. The seventh offers an analytic framework which a) organizes the delivery of treatment and helps in prevention, b) provides institutions and government as the basis for public policy, c) gains financial backing from insurance companies, d) challenges the criminal justice system to better understand and care for pathological gamblers, e) gives theoretical, empirical, and clinical support to GA and the state and federal gambling councils, and f) shapes public opinion and public expectations. The eighth strategy outlines the procedures for treatment: a) assessment, b) diagnosis, c) treatment planning, d) ongoing evaluation and modification of treatment plan, e) prognosis, and f) follow-up. The ninth defines pathological gambling according to DSM criteria. Pathological gambling begins and ends with the DSM. The tenth further supports the DSM diagnosis by getting rid of the necessity for etiology. The eleventh pursues research that provides averages, means, and generalizations rather than differences and uniqueness. The twelfth searches for predictive validity in diagnosis and treatment. The thirteenth only considers issues of context—such as gender, age, ethnicity, class, occupation, family background, friends and current family dynamics, economics, politics and culture—after the diagnosis is established. And, finally, the fourteenth outlines a framework that is linear, rational, and empirically reductionistic and positivistic.

Blume's definition of the content and process of medical treatment is not based on any one particular strategy or statement, such as the search for a biological basis to gambling or the use of medical professionals in treatment. Instead, it emerges out of the combined effect fourteen different, yet similar, intersecting strategies have on one another. In this way Blume's definition is an improvement over our original working definition by Conrad and Schneider (1980). Blume's definition helps us better understand the discursive complexity of gambling treatment. It reveals that gambling treatment is not a static, conceptual structure which refers, in "dictionary-like" terms, to a specific once and for all, never to change, discursive practice. It is something entirely different, something which cannot be reduced to a structure, discourse, interaction, or technique or style of treatment. Instead, it is something which I call an organizing practice (Castellani 1999).

The Medical Model as Organizing Practice

Organizing practice provides a framework for the study of gambling treatment. It conceptualizes treatment as a two-fold set of discursive inter-actions. First, there are the interactions between the fourteen discursive strategies Blume (1987) outlined for us. These strategies profile the discursive context through which treatment takes place. Second, there are the interactions these fourteen strategies have with the agents involved in their practice. Agents range from clinicians and pathological gamblers to professions and organizations such as the field of addiction treatment and research. Blume's fourteen discursive strategies are defined as discourse in practice as interaction, and the inter-acting agents who use them are defined as inter-action in practice as discourse.

Each of these definitions represents one fold of the two-fold interactive process of organizing practice. It is important to understand that neither is the basis for the other. They both create and influence one another. They are each other. Therefore, when we point to the content and process of gambling treatment, we are referring to the result of these complex discursive interactions; that is, we are referring to the inter-actions between discursive strategies and discursive agents.

But that is not the end. Intersecting with these discursive interactions are another set of practices which define the socio-historical terms and conditions of gambling treatment. The terms and conditions of gambling treatment initially include a) the field of gambling research and treatment, b) the field of addiction research and treatment, c) the changing health care system, and d) Gamblers Anonymous and its members. They also additionally include a) the criminal justice system, b) the gambling industry, c) state and federal government, d) pathological gamblers and their families, e) the gambling councils, and f) our contemporary gambling culture.

Just like the medical model, each of these terms and conditions are their own organizing practice: they are comprised of their own two-fold interactive process and emerge out of a complex series of discursive interactions. While separate, what brings them together is the socio-historical manner in which they intersect with the content and process of gambling treatment. It is, therefore, out of the interaction between the content and process of medical treatment, as they intersect with the practices which define their terms and conditions, that the organizing practice of the medical model of gambling treatment emerges.

For example, when Custer created the content and process of medical treatment, he did so by borrowing the techniques and tools of addiction treatment in general. As a discursive interaction, he and his colleagues inter-acted with the discursive strategies of alcohol treatment to make a new organizing practice called the medical model of gambling treatment. But, when Custer engaged in these discursive interactions, he did so within a certain set of historical terms and conditions. He was working for the

United States Government at an in-patient Veterans Administration (VA) addiction treatment facility, which, at the time, had lots of money for new therapies. He was therefore able to do almost whatever he wanted. It is certainly not the same today in an era when treatment programs are being shut down left and right. Terms and conditions influence content and process, and vice versa.

The resulting discursive order that emerges from the complex discursive inter-actions that Custer and others engaged in is defined as a *negotiated order.* The organizing practice of gambling treatment is a negotiated order. It is a negotiated order because the intersection of its complex discursive inter-actions can only take place through the process of discursive negotiation. For example, as therapists throughout the United States practice the medical model of gambling treatment, they do so by negotiating their practices into the worlds of addiction treatment, health care, and mental health. As an exercised discursive framework, as a practiced-sign-in-interaction, the medical model must be *exercised* to be useful; agents have to put it into practice for it to exist. Its essential structure is defined only because it exists within the world. As an organizing practice, gambling treatment cannot exist outside of time or space. It is not an ahistorical, static framework which is somehow applied to life. Therapists do not simply apply the medical model to gambling. They make it part of everything else they do. Thus, like the rest of life, the medical model of gambling treatment is always, already (in Heideggerian terms) within-the-world: within time, within space, within history, within society, within the individual.

Because it is within the world, the medical model of gambling treatment is always already making a history of its own within a discursive history not of its own making. In other words, because there are so many different countervailing discursive inter-actions taking place at any given moment in time, the medical model of gambling treatment can only influence the larger and smaller fields in which it is practiced—such as the field of addiction treatment and the changing health care system—by somehow negotiating its ways into the currently existing practices that are already taking place.

The reverse it also true. Therapists and treatment facilities can only negotiate the medical model into the larger and smaller fields of discursive practice because these practices, such as the health care system, always already have some level of discursive space to accommodate them, no matter how dominating a particular set of negotiated relations happen to be. And so, the field of treatment and the larger and smaller systems through which it takes place are always already a series of negotiated orders. In other words, to enter into this exercised discursive fray, accommodations and alterations must be made. The medical model doesn't simply replace the preceding set of discursive practices. Instead, it integrates itself into what currently exists and thereby influences change through negotiation. Without accommodation on the part of what currently exists, negotiation could never take place and change would never happen.

The concept of organizing practice as a negotiated order does not, however, dismiss the inequality of negotiation; it only points to the process by which discursive interaction takes place. The discursive interactions comprising the content and process of medical work, as well as its terms and conditions, are not in balance with one another. The negotiations by which they are created are imbalanced as well. Patients and clinicians don't have the same level of power, neither do treatment experts and the organizations for which they work. As such, domination, exploitation, and oppression are always present. But, they are only present as conditional states of the more basic negotiated order they create and are created by. The influence of the changing health care system on gambling treatment, for example, has changed over time. Over the past decade it has increased in control, making the discursive negotiations of gambling treatment more difficult. But, in response, treatment has become hyper-medicalized by focusing its research on the biological, thereby making a stronger case for the utility of treatment. It is because of the constant negotiated nature of inter-action that freedom is a necessary condition of organizing practice.

However, because we are in negotiation, we are also never completely free. We are always, in some way, controlled. Negotiation represents difference and spacing in our discursive relations with one another, and yet negotiation is constraining and ordering because we can never escape our being in the world, our being in inter-action (even when alone); we are never free of the inter-act of negotiation itself. We are always within the world creating and being created by the two-fold interactive process of organizing practice. Despite degrees of freedom, because gambling treatment experts are within the world, they always have to negotiate their position. In the 1970s it was easier; in the 1990s it is more difficult. Either way, they are in negotiation and so are never free to simply do as they please. From this perspective, power is a negotiated process.

To understand better the negotiated nature of the medical model of gambling treatment, even within states of domination, let us return again to the two-fold interactive process of organizing practice.

As stated, one half of the two-fold interactive process is the interactions between discursive strategies. Discursive strategies replace the traditional concept of social structure. In organizing practice there are no structures, only discourses in interaction as practice. In place of the search for structures, the discursive interactionist looks for nexus points: those points of intersection where a competing set of strategies come together to form the practice being studied. Once a nexus point is determined, the researcher focuses on the discursive strategies defining a given practice. The focus is never on any one strategy. Discursive order emerges through the practice of discursive strategies in inter-action with one another, as they come together to form a particular nexus point.

Blume's definition of the medical model provides one such nexus point. The content and process of the medical model is the intersection of fourteen similar yet different discursive strategies. These discursive strategies, as they form the content and process of the medical model, intersect with the discursive strategies comprising the terms and conditions of gambling treatment. For example, the changing health care system is comprised of the discursive strategies of the medical profession and its internal dynamics, corporate purchasers and buyers, other allied health professionals, state and federal level government, and so on. All of these intersecting strategies influence the strategies defined as the content and process of medical work. This intersection is evidenced by Blume's (1987) statement that "[t]he medical model encourages the development and financial support of resources to help pathological gamblers and their families, and. . . . provides a framework for enlightened public policy in the regulation of the gambling industry, and for rational approaches to social and legal problems related to the disease" (p. 244). Certainly, the medical model was not constructed to obtain political and economic support. But, as a set of discursive strategies, it negotiates well with the discursive strategies of the changing health care system and government and is thereby able to gain a certain level of power. As used by specific agents in response to specific problems, the discursive strategies of the medical model can influence government and the changing health care system to respond favorably.

And so, like organizing practice, discursive strategies do not exist outside of time and space, they do not exist outside of practice, and they do not exist outside of inter-action, that is, their shared relationship with one another. Discursive strategies are practiced inter-actions, one strategy with another. They do not exist on their own. Their power is dependent upon their ability, as strategies, to negotiate their situations. The medical model is comprised of a series of inter-connecting discursive strategies, all in practiced inter-action with one another. Without these fourteen strategies intersecting with the terms and conditions of their practice, the medical model would not exist.

But, the power obtained through discursive strategy is not specific enough to accomplish any particular agenda. Because discursive strategies are practiced within-the-world they are intentional, but their intentionality is nonsubjective. Take, for example, strategies three through five. Strategy three situates pathological gambling within the theoretical and clinical jurisdiction of the medical model. Strategy four defines and treats it as a disease, a medical condition, a mental illness. And strategy five transfers the tools, techniques and theoretical devices of the medical model onto the problems of gambling. Each of these strategies are intended toward the care of gamblers. But, as a general set of strategies, they are without agency. We need the other half of the two-fold interactive process to provide that information. On their own, discursive strategies organize the general set of intentions through which gambling treatment takes place, and in so doing negotiate a series of power relations, but they do so without a positing subject.

Strategy six makes this clear. Strategy six enforces the act of hiring professionals to do treatment, not just physicians, but psychiatric nurses, clinical psychologists, social workers, and certified addiction specialists as well. But, which physicians and which nurses? Do they mean Custer, Lesieur or Blume, or someone entirely different? These agents are vital to the content and process of gambling treatment and its negotiations with its terms and conditions. Relying upon Blume's outline of discursive strategy alone we therefore do not arrive at this subjectified dimension of the history of gambling treatment.

Nevertheless, the strength of discursive strategies is the power of discursive influence they enforce. Those that do treatment are professionals; gambling is practiced as a disease; its problems are located in the body; the tools and techniques of the medical model must be used, and treatment takes place within the jurisdiction of the medical field. Furthermore, those who are treated must be diagnosed as pathological gamblers; they must fit the criteria of the DSM, and they are to be treated according to a rather specific treatment protocol: a) assessment, b) diagnosis, c) treatment planning, d) ongoing evaluation and modification of treatment plan, e) prognosis, and f) follow-up. The content and process of medical treatment is, therefore, very well organized by its discursive strategies. They provide the general discursive intentionality by which treatment takes place. But, as I said, they are nonsubjective. Subjectivity comes through the second fold of the two-fold interactive process.

The second set of discursive interactions are between inter-acting agents as they inter-act with themselves, each other, and the interacting strategies of the medical model of gambling treatment. These inter-actions are defined as inter-action in practice as discourse. From this definition, agents are broadly conceptualized as individuals, groups, families, institutions, organizations, professions, cultures, states, nations and everything in-between. The intentional and subjectified inter-actions between discursive agents integrate both the content and process of gambling treatment as well as its terms and conditions.

According to the concept of organizing practice, agency is not defined as the singular actions of any particular individual. Instead, the focus is on agents in inter-action. We are within the world; we are, therefore, within inter-action. Discursive interactions do not start with the individual and then proceed to the larger social reality. Neither do they start with discursive strategies and proceed inward. Instead, they start right in the middle of inter-action itself. In terms of discursive agents, the focus is on the interactions between them. Agents do not float around separate from the intersecting organizing practices within which they exist. They both make them up and are made by them, and they are made through their interactions with one another as well. Gambling treatment did not start with Custer and proceed to the rest of the country, nor did it start with the rest of the country and proceed to Custer. It took place within the discursive interactions between Custer and his colleagues and the discursive strategies within which they existed.

Let's approach this discussion from another direction. Typically, though not always, we think of structures, like the medical model, as a backdrop for a particular set of interactions—even when created by the interactions between individuals. As a backdrop, these structures are conceptualized as relatively static and stable, changing only seldom and very slowly. From this perspective, often the objective of research is to define what a particular structure is (e.g., "the medical model is that which locates the source of deviant behavior within the individual," Conrad and Schneider 1980, p. 64). With this definition, researchers then move on to explore how people exist within and carry out these structures, such as therapists and patients.

From this perspective, therapy appears to take place within the structure of medical treatment. The structure of the medical model, as a form of power, conditions and constrains how treatment takes place. Therapists and patients are not seen in terms of how they influence these structures, but are instead studied in terms of how they carry them out. In other words, patients and therapists come to the "truth" about their subjectivity by positioning themselves in relation to a particular set of already existing prescriptive codes. And so, they are implicated in these structures only insomuch as they determine their conduct according to the rules governing their behavior. Therapists and patients are typically seen as the vehicle and outcome of the processes of structure—even in micro interactionist terms—but are often not seen as the cause.

For example, given the constraints of the medical model, a researcher may examine how therapists impose upon patients a certain way of being that dominates their understandings of themselves; that is, how they construct the "truth" about their subjectivity as a pathological gambler. Patients are then studied to see how they resist these constraining structures, how they make for themselves a sense of self or existence that counteracts the structures imposed upon them—a pathological gambler may decided to gamble on some level even though he's been told that abstinence is the only viable way to recovery. In these types of studies, structure is a given. How therapists and patients are involved in the act of structure itself, how they both create and are created by it through the inter-actions they define as their lives is not really questioned. These types of analyses therefore give the impression that the medical model goes on behind the backs of people, like the change of scenery in a play.

The concept of organizing practice takes us away from these types of research questions. Discursive agency is conceptualized as something entirely different. It is conceptualized as the creation and enactment of discourse through interaction. Discursive agents are the cause, vehicle, and effect of discursive strategy.

Think about it. Without discursive agency, discursive strategies would never inter-act. The easiest example, as I have already illustrated above through the activities of Custer and his colleagues, is the intersection between the content and process of gambling treatment and its terms and conditions. The content and process of medical treatment is the act of care itself. But, who is doing this treatment? Discursive agents, that's who—therapists, treatment centers, the field of gambling treatment. Likewise, there are the terms and conditions within which medical work takes place. Again, who is involved in these discursive strategies? The same discursive agents.

The importance of discursive agents is that they cannot be reduced to the power and influence of any one particular set of organizing practices and their accompanying discursive strategies. Agents are always already more than that. They are always already within the intersection between the discursive strategies of several intersecting organizing practices. In other words, organizing practices, such as the medical model of gambling treatment, come into existence always already negotiating their way into a set of existing organizing practices, such as the changing health care system, but only because agents are already involved in these existing discursive strategies. It is by and through them that the new sets of practices find their way. Agents, such as Custer, Lesieur, Rosenthal, and Rugle created the new organizing practices of gambling treatment and they integrated them with others, such as their respective professional backgrounds (e.g., psychiatry, sociology, psychiatry and clinical psychology). As discursive agents, Custer and colleagues were the cause, vehicle, and effect of the discursive strategies in which they engaged. It was through their efforts that the power and influence of the fourteen strategies of the medical model of gambling treatment had their effect.

As such, discursive agents such as Custer and his colleagues provide the subjectified intentionality of discursive practice. Through their interactions with the discursive strategies in which they exist, gambling treatment programs throughout the United States make the medical model their own. In other words, treatment is something we do. People go to school to learn how to do therapy. They put together for themselves a toolbox of techniques which they gain by studying different models of treatment, by putting these models into practice with different patients, and then deciding for themselves what they like, while discarding the rest. Therapists and treatment professionals, like all of us, are influenced by trends. They are influenced by the latest jargon and procedures considered *en vogue* at the time of their training. They don't just simply enact these discourses, they use them as they see fit. They try them on for size, make them accomodate their own biases and opinions about what health is, what pathology is, and what constitutes in their mind the best way to care for someone else. Then they go out and get a job. They work for an out-patient gambling treatment program or an in-patient treatment center. There they run into psychiatric nurses, social workers, physician assistants, clinical psychologists, certified addiction specialists, psychiatrists, and others—all of whom also went to school, learned how to do therapy according to their various traditions, and decided for themselves what constituted good gambling treatment.

The interactions all of these different professionals have with one another are also influenced by differences between individuals. Some people are extroverted, others are more reserved. One person is healthier than another, or simply better at doing therapy. On top of this are differences in gender, ethnicity, class, social upbringing, family of origin and so on. All of these differences make for different ways of doing therapy. Women in the gambling treatment field may be more sensitive to the issues of family and use the medical model in a less paternalistic manner. Treatment professionals who've recovered from the experiences of pathological gambling will have different insights than those who've never gambled. These all make for differences.

Further still are the differences in institutional organization and location. Institutions and organization have their own set of rules and procedures, their own hierarchy of values. Treatment programs have their own therapeutic agendas. Some treatment centers use the twelve-step approach of Gamblers Anonymous as their guideline; others are more humanistic, while others follow a particular therapeutic style. Just as individuals are raised within certain traditions of therapy, so are treatment facilities. The people who run a group practice, a counseling center, or an in-patient treatment program write up their own guidelines for treatment. They define the length of stay, the duration of treatment, how much treatment will be given, the daily schedule of patients, the amount of time therapists spend with patients, the payment schedule, lunch breaks, weekend passes for patients and so on. These all represent variation in the way Blume's fourteen strategies are practiced and so introduce variation in the level of control and power the discursive strategies of the medical model exercise in their interactions with other practices.

Again, this is further complicated by changes in the political, cultural, and economic arrangement of mental health itself. As the larger health care system changes, so does treatment. As I pointed out above, at certain points in the history of mental health, more money has been available for treatment. We are currently in very difficult times financially and politically. Culture and politics change as well. They too influence how treatment is done. We went through a period where psychiatry ruled the treatment of addiction. Now social workers and nurses run the show. Things change.

Even with this brief outline, our picture of how the discursive strategies of the medical model of gambling treatment are practiced is definitely more complex. You have individuals, institutions, cultures, politics, economics, the changing health care system, differences between and within professions and so on, all interacting with one another to define the organizing practice we call the medical model of gambling treatment.

As such, the interactions between discursive agents and the strategies of which they are a part are, as I've said several times now, a negotiated order. It is open-ended, incomplete, dynamic and in process. Despite its stability, it is always changing. How it exists in one location may be different from the next. Medical treatment in Ohio differs from treatment in Florida and Minnesota. And yet, because of the practices which organize it, there are similarities and consistencies across all of these different locations. The "medical model of gambling treatment" is therefore a heading which we use to describe a way of inter-acting that is the basis for the act of gambling treatment. It informs our understanding of pathological gambling as much as it is a form we apply to understand.

Given the complexities of the two-fold interactive process, the study of organizing practice (which we engage in through the method of assemblage) must always situate itself in the (in)-between of things: between the inter-actions of discourse and agency, between the inter-actions of researchers and that which is researched, between practiced discourses in inter-action, and between discursive agents in inter-action. Organizing practice is always already within inter-action. As such, it is as an inter-active, analytic framework for the study of the (in)-between of negotiated symbolic (discursive) reality.

Given this general orientation, organizing practice is defined as: *discourse in practice as interaction and inter-action in practice as discourse* (Castellani 1998). Organizing practice overcomes distinctions between text and life, discourse and inter-action, knowledge and social context, agency and structure. It is a sign-in-practice. As a practiced sign, the exercise of organizing practice orders how we care for ourselves and others according to the numerous discursive frameworks we put into practice daily. Discourse and inter-action are never separated. Discourse is practiced inter-action and inter-action is practiced discourse.

In summary, then, as an organizing practice, gambling treatment is a two-fold, inter-active, negotiated order, which is comprised of a complex series of inter-actions between and within discursive strategies and between and within inter-acting agents as they interact with each other, themselves, and the inter-acting discursive strategies within which they exist. These inter-actions, both within and between the two-fold exercise of organizing practice, require constant negotiation. As such, the medical model of gambling treatment, as an organizing practice, is never complete.

Custer and the Medical Model of Gambling Treatment

Our assemblage of pathological gambling as organizing practice continues now with Custer's creation of the Brecksville Gambling Treatment Program. Our goal here is to add yet another layer to our history by examining the relationship Custer, as a single individual, had with the larger history of which he was a part. We do this in an attempt to show that the interactions of a single individual can change history even though that individual, in this case Custer, a) is not the beginning or end of the inter-actions involved in this history; b) is not entirely aware of his involvement in this history beyond his own subjective intentions; and c) is influencing and influenced by the larger history of which he is a part, through his negotiation of the organizing practices in which he finds himself—as such there is no micro/macro analysis here, only the study of inter-action in practice as discourse.

As Robert Custer stated, "The story starts in April 1971" when he was the "director of the alcoholism-treatment program at the Veterans Administration Hospital in Brecksville, Ohio" (Custer and Milt 1985 p. 216). Custer was approached by several members of a local GA group concerned about some of their members whose problems, they felt, went beyond the expertise of GA. These people required professional treatment. At the time, Custer had only vaguely heard of pathological gambling. The only theory explaining pathological gambling, although quite marginal at the time, was psychoanalytic. The theory was Bergler's. Although he didn't have a theory of his own, Custer somehow disagreed: "To me," he stated, "compulsive gambling appeared to be a disorder of impulse control, and I believed that any treatment that was devised would have to approach it from that position. But we had nothing to go on" (p. 217). Custer would have to start from scratch. But, he was not without his hunches: "I knew, in advance, that Gamblers Anonymous was patterned after Alcoholics Anonymous, and I knew about AA and its program intimately because of my work with alcoholics. On that basis, I was prepared for the similarities" (p. 217).

To familiarize himself with the problem, Custer attended several GA meetings and met regularly with GA members to discuss the problems of gambling. What hit him after only a couple of meetings was the striking similarity between alcoholism and pathological gambling. He stated: "I saw desperate people, in great pain, suffering, helpless and hopeless, and, from a psychiatric standpoint, these were people we would regard as emergencies" (Custer and Milt 1985, p. 217).

Already, we see Custer engaging in discursive negotiation with the phenomena he was observing. He was grounded in the discursive strategies of psychiatry and in-patient addiction treatment. Even his terminology was medical: these patients were "emergencies." It is within these practices, as he himself negotiated and interpreted them, that he viewed the world. We wouldn't expect the process to be any different. As such, the medical model was his practiced discursive standpoint. From his first meeting with GA members, he began to modify his understanding of addiction in application to pathological gambling. As stated by him, he viewed gambling from a "psychiatric standpoint."

Interestingly enough, Custer didn't engage in these negotiations alone. He was in inter-action with GA members who already believed, themselves, that pathological gambling fit within the discursive practices of the medical model. In other words, Custer didn't go out looking for the problem. It was brought to him personally by members of GA who wanted to know if he "could start an institutional program there at the hospital for the treatment of compulsive gamblers, similar to the one [he] had for alcoholics" (Custer and Milt 1985, p. 217). And so, from the beginning, Custer formed his ideas about gambling in discursive inter-action. The content and process were already merging with its terms and conditions.

In terms of the terms and conditions influencing this initial process, you have two primary sets of organizing practice intersecting one another.

On one hand, you have the practices of the members of Gamblers Anonymous, which include the twelve-Steps and an implicit set of practices linked with the medical model through Alcoholics Anonymous, which GA is patterned after. And on the other, you have the practices Custer brought to these interactions: the field of addiction treatment and research, the practices of psychiatry and the medical model, and the organizing practice of the health care system and the federal government, which at the time offered the financial and political support for the expansion of medical treatment and knowledge.

Given our understanding of the two-fold inter-active process, we know that these two inter-secting practices did not simply collide to form a new practice which would become the content and process of gambling treatment. Nor did the medical model easily impose upon pathological gambling a new dominating set of discursive strategies. A more complex and subtle process was taking place, a process which required a series of negotiations by both sets of discursive agents.

Remember, discursive strategies are intentional but nonsubjective. In the case of GA, its discursive strategies were only designed to care for pathological gamblers. The intentions became specific only as these GA agents, in inter-action with one another, subjectified these strategies for a particular end. In this case, the specific subjectified intentionality was directed toward the establishment of an in-patient gambling treatment program. In 1971, in Ohio, GA members made accommodations to their practices in order to achieve treatment.

Likewise, the medical model and its sub-practices—psychiatry and addiction treatment—were deliberately designed to care for people with drug and alcohol problems. The intention was the application of these strategies to those types of problems. But, there was no specific goal to establish and legitimate yet another area of care. Insomuch as the discursive strategies of the medical model came to dominate the care of pathological gamblers, it was non-intentional. The intentionality came from Custer and his associates. They purposed the medical model toward the treatment of pathological gambling and made the modifications necessary. And so, while a history was taking place which was larger than Custer and his colleagues, it was dependent upon their specific intentions.

As these agents and their practices came together, a number of negotiations took place. The members of GA had to work out for themselves what medical treatment would mean and how it would influence their lives, and Custer had to determine how he would reconstruct his psychiatric framework in application to gambling. A precedent was set. Alcoholics Anonymous had adopted the medical model a long time ago. Gamblers Anonymous had followed in the footsteps of AA up to this point, people with alcoholism went to treatment, so why shouldn't such a program exist for pathological gamblers? As practiced in the lives of these people, it made perfect discursive sense. And so Custer came to what was to him and the members of GA the next logical conclusion: "If the basic AA program could work for gamblers, why would not the treatment program we used at the hospital for alcoholics also work to treat compulsive gamblers" (Custer and Milt 1985 p. 218)?

Thus, by 1972, the first in-patient treatment program for pathological gambling was started. Custer stated: "My associate Alida Glen, Ph.D., and I designed a treatment program patterned after the one we were using to treat alcoholics. [Starting with that as our tentative premise, we were on our way]" (Custer and Milt 1985, p. 218).

Custer's strategy for gambling treatment mimicked the treatment approach he and his staff used for alcoholics at the Brecksville Veterans Addiction Recovery Center. His protocol followed Blume's fourteen strategies of treatment, minus the usage of the DSM diagnosis of pathological gambling (strategies nine and ten) since it wasn't published until 1980. We will now explore how Custer negotiated his interaction with these twelve discursive strategies.

First of all, the individual gambler was defined as the focus of treatment (strategy one). The gambler came in for treatment; the gambler went to therapy; the gambler went to evening groups; the gambler made a treatment plan; the gambler learned about his problems; and the gambler was the focus of recovery. Issues of social context (strategy thirteen)—including gender, age, ethnicity, class, occupation, economics, politics and culture—were secondary, if even considered. For example, Custer didn't contemplate why pathological gambling was a disease that plagued more men than women, or why most gamblers were white, or why, as the 1980s progressed, it attacked the middle-class. These types of questions weren't within the purview of the discursive strategies in which he was raised. He was educated, as a psychiatrist, in the standard approach to treatment, which has always focused on the individual at the expense of the social. Within Custer's discursive framework, the dualism between the individual and the social remained firmly entrenched.

The limitation to Custer's individualism was his inability to successfully negotiate some of the more important terms and conditions in which the Brecksville Gambling Treatment Program took place. Specifically, he could not address how the social context of patients influenced their recovery. This profound limitation was also the result of strategies eleven, twelve and fourteen. Treatment leaned toward: a) averages, means and generalizations rather than differences and uniqueness; b) the search for predictive validity in diagnosis and treatment; and c) a belief in a linear, rational, and empirically reductionistic and positivistic approach to causality. And so, while Custer's construction of gambling treatment successfully navigated the negotiated difficulties surrounding the establishment of the treatment program itself, the terms and conditions of patients coming in for treatment were met with less success (this remains a major problem, even today, in almost every gambling treatment unit throughout the country).

Nevertheless, despite Custer's highly individualistic approach to treatment, he was unique (and still is) in his emphasis on the family: "We realized early that even with the best therapy, the gambling addict would find it very difficult, perhaps impossible, to achieve recovery alone. The family, we realized, plays an immensely important part" (Custer and Milt 1985, p. 224). Custer designed the treatment program to include individual counseling for spouses and, toward the end of treatment, offered cojoint therapy for the gambler and his spouse if they wanted it. Still, even with the family as a focus, it was primarily in relation to the gambler. The goal of treatment, as Custer stated, was to "enable the patient to stop gambling" (p. 224). The involvement of family and friends was only in relation to this goal. If the gambler relapsed, therapy with the family ended.

Moving along, the next thing Custer did was to locate the sources of pathological gambling in origins other than the gambling itself (strategy two). Custer stated: "Certainly, we were going to continue to deal with the gambling, per se, trying to motivate the patient to give up gambling, to get his gambling under control" (Custer and Milt 1985, p. 221). "But," argued Custer, "right along with that we had to deal with the personality and behavior problems—the dishonesty, impatience, intolerance and manipulation, inability to plan and make decisions, avoidance of responsibility, insensitivity to the feelings and needs of others, poor problem-solving ability" (p. 221). All of these various "other" problems, which became the focus of treatment, were the "real" problems according to Custer. Defined in medical terms, these problems were consistent with the focus of gambling research (which we reviewed in chapter three): impulsivity and emotional problems (impatience and intolerance), attention deficits (inability to plan and make decisions, poor problem-solving ability), and personality disorders and problems with relationships (manipulation, insensitivity to the feelings and needs of others).

Third, Custer defined treatment on an in-patient basis and made the gambling treatment program part of the larger Veterans Addiction Recovery Center. In so doing, Custer not only located pathological gambling within the theoretical and clinical jurisdiction of the medical model (strategy three), he transferred the tools, techniques, and theoretical devices of the medical model onto the problems of gambling itself (strategy five). In other words, by simply locating the treatment of gambling within the physical confines of the Veterans Administration hospital, Custer made the treatment of pathological gambling *medical* in both its content (the tools and techniques) and its process (the flow of treatment itself, from detoxification and assessment to individual and group therapy and follow-up treatment).

Part of locating his treatment program in the VA included hiring professional healers. The house staff Custer hired followed strategy six. They were not just physicians, but "a professional psychiatrist, psychologist, social worker [and] nurse" to be exact (Custer and Milt 1985, p. 218).

Next, Custer defined pathological gambling as a disease (strategy four). Custer made several statements on this issue. "Compulsive gambling—or 'pathological gambling,' as it is called in professional terms—is an illness, a psychological illness" (Custer and Milt 1985, p. 36). While the research has yet to conclusively show pathological gambling as such, "there is agreement on this, at least . . . that it is a psychological illness with psychological causes, and that it is possible to treat it and to bring about recovery" (p. 36). "In other words," argued Custer, "pathological gambling has now been recognized as an illness by the professions authorized to make this sort of judgement" (p. 36). Through these statements Custer made a number of important discursive negotiations that helped him deal with the terms and conditions within which he grounded the content and process of gambling treatment. His argument was primarily based on professional authority. The fact that treatment was offered by professional practitioners in a legitimate in-patient treatment center, that was recognized by the government, made pathological gambling a legitimate disease of the mind.

These are important words. It is necessary to understand that while Custer appropriated pathological gambling into the field of addiction treatment, its legitimacy was not guaranteed. In fact, the larger field of addiction treatment didn't immediately embrace the idea. And so, while Custer brought pathological gambling into addiction treatment and the medical model, once back in the fold he still had a lot of convincing to do. Arguing that pathological gambling was a legitimate mental illness helped him in his negotiations. It elevated gambling to the level of addictive disease.

Again, this reveals the nonsubjective aspects of discursive intentionality. While the twelve strategies defining the content and process of medical treatment were constructed to care for people, the question of whether they were specifically intended for the treatment of pathological gambling was open to negotiation. To make pathological gambling a medical disorder, subjective intentionality was necessary. Some level of agency had to do the research, do the treatment, and go out and convince others. It is for this reason that the work of Custer and his colleagues focused on apologetics as much as understanding. They were working hard to persuade the larger fields of practices within which they were operating that their medical designation should be accepted as such. It is for this same reason that Blume (1987) argued in her article that the medical model (strategy seven) offers an analytic framework which not only organizes the delivery of treatment and help in prevention, but also provides institutions and government the basis for private and public policy, gains financial backing from insurance companies, and shapes professional opinion and expectations.

The fifth thing Custer did was to put into practice the process of treatment itself (strategy eight). Treatment was comprised of six basic elements. First and foremost was group therapy. Custer stated: "We decided that the most effective way to take on this rather formidable task, and to affect some basic changes in the remaining time we had left, would be to concentrate most of our efforts on group therapy" (Custer and Milt 1985, p. 221). Group provided an open forum for patients to inter-act. Custer understood they knew each other better than staff anyway, and, since most of the gambler's problems were in their relationships, it was a chance for them to really work on their problems. In addition to group therapy, gamblers received individual counseling. And, if their spouses were willing, they too could receive a few individual sessions themselves. Custer knew the family members of these gamblers were angry and confused. Putting them immediately in a session with the gambler would only prove disastrous.

So, first they were seen separately, and then, toward the end of treatment, if they were both willing, they saw a therapist together. Gamblers also attended relaxation classes and recreational therapy to help them deal with their boredom. One of the biggest complaints of gamblers once they stopped gambling was that they were bored. The thing they enjoyed most in life had been taken away. It was important, therefore, to teach them other things to do with their time. In addition to therapy, gamblers attended nightly GA meetings and put together a follow-up plan and a schedule of GA meetings to attend once they completed treatment.

These, then, were the twelve discursive strategies Custer negotiated to start the first in-patient gambling treatment program in the United States. In fact, during his tenure at the Brecksville program, Custer and his colleagues deviated little from the medical model they initially implemented. As the 1970s and 1980s progressed, Custer's treatment regime solidified and became a standard approach to gambling treatment throughout the country. In fact, it influenced the establishment of several Veterans Administration Gambling Treatment Programs—one in Brooklyn, Miami, New Jersey and California—as well as the South Oaks Hospital in Long Island and the Compulsive Gambling Center Inc., run by Dr. Lorenz in Maryland.

As this brief history of the Brecksville Gambling Treatment Program has revealed, through his interactions, Custer proved to be a rather excellent discursive agent. But, as we have learned, he was not alone. He had the interactive support of several important discursive practices and agents, including the field of addiction treatment, the medical model, the disease concept, local GA members, the federal institution for which he worked, and a political, economic and health care climate that gave him the negotiated space to accomplish his task. Thus, as a moment in the history of pathological gambling, the establishment of the Brecksville Gambling Treatment Program was a truly remarkable discursive feat.

Chapter 6

GAMBLERS ANONYMOUS AND THE GAMBLING COUNCILS

Throughout the 1980s and 1990s, in-patient gambling treatment centers such as the Brecksville program, had an immense impact on the thinking of members of Gamblers Anonymous (GA) and the various major state and national gambling councils across the United States. The impact was such that the fourteen discursive strategies of the medical model became the primary practice used by the councils and various members of GA to accomplish their agendas.

The Start of GA and the National Council

The same year Bergler was writing his classic text, two men, tired of making the same mistakes over and over again, got together. The year was 1957. The place: Los Angeles, California, the land of gambling, the last frontier. These two anonymous men decided to form a partnership. They wanted to put an end to their gambling, their excesses, their problems. Success! They actually stopped gambling. This gave them courage, courage to form the first Gamblers Anonymous meeting. The meeting was held on 13 September 1957. From there things progressed.

The history of Gambler Anonymous is different from AA, its predecessor. Prohibition ended in 1933, so by the time AA caught on, drinking was already a national "past time"—people understood the problems associated with drinking. GA was different. Because gambling was illegal until the 1970s, GA took a longer time to gain acceptance. It was hard for people to accept pathological gambling as a disease. Once the problems of gambling hit the middle-class, however, things changed. GA's recognition started to improve. More meetings were held throughout the country. Around the same time, the National Council on Problem Gambling was established.[1]

Rosecrance (1985a) explains that the National Council on Compulsive Gambling—which recently changed its name to the National Council on Problem Gambling to be more inclusive—was formed when several members of Gamblers Anonymous got together with Monsignor Joseph Dunne to address the problems of pathological gambling on a national scale. Several lawyers and medical experts were also asked to help, one of whom was Robert Custer.

Historically, the discursive practices of GA were intentionally constructed to avoid conflict with the larger political and social and historical terms and conditions within which it was exercised. As a set of practices, the intention was toward recovering gamblers. By the 1970s, however, certain members of GA realized that neither the government nor the social sciences were going to do much to educate or treat the nation. The problems of pathological gambling were increasing. So, these subjectified agents decided to do something, which is when they ran into Monsignor Dunne.

Dunne was working with the New York City Police at the time dealing with alcoholism on the police force. Dunne quickly noticed that the men he was counseling also had gambling problems. Dunne got involved with Gamblers Anonymous and began discussing the possibility of putting together a national council. The National Council on Problem Gambling was officially established in 1972. Since then, the Council has worked hard to increase national awareness about gambling, and they've served as a lobby for the medical model "by sponsoring research and funding projects that advance the illness concept (Hyde, 1978: 48–9)" (Rosecrance 1985a, p. 278). They've also published a newsletter to keep their members informed of developments in the field of compulsive gambling, and they've been the primary funding source for the one and only journal devoted to the topic of problem and pathological gambling, *The Journal of Gambling Studies*. The current President of the National Council is attorney, Paul Ash, who also works with the Florida Council on Compulsive Gambling. In addition to the National Council, there are thirty two state level affiliate councils.

GA's Acknowledgment of the Disease Model

Historically, the members of Gamblers Anonymous have hardly been passive recipients of the practices of the medical model. In fact, over its forty-year history, GA members have actively sought a role in integrating into their lives the discursive strategies of the medical model and its treatment. They are responsible for establishing both the first in-patient treatment program and for starting a national council. And, they've been involved in the treatment process, from working as part of the treatment staff to providing evening meetings. The heavily integrated inter-action of GA and the medical model is a picture of discursive negotiation at its best.

Take a look at a survey done by Julian Taber, a one-time member of the Brecksville program and recognized leading scholar. It illustrates clearly how integrated the medical model and Gamblers Anonymous are. Taber's survey was published in GA's *Sharing Recovery Through Gamblers Anonymous* (1984). The survey was completed by a sample of GA members, treatment experts, psychologists and psychiatrists. The first set of questions pertain to the theoretical and conceptual understanding of pathological gambling.

When asked if they thought it was appropriate to view pathological gambling as a disease or disorder, 96 percent of the GA members surveyed agreed, 90 percent of treatment experts agreed, 62 percent of psychologists agreed, and 75 percent of all psychiatrists agreed. Since psychiatrists and GA members have the most to gain from the medical model, it would be expected that they would have the highest percentages. Psychologists are somewhat more resistant to a straightforward medical model because of their desire to defend their own disciplinary and professional boundaries. Overall, the total percentages were quite high.

When asked if pathological gambling is probably an addiction similar in nature to other addictions such as drugs and alcohol, 91 percent of all GA members agreed, followed by 83 percent of all treatment experts, 88 percent of all psychologists, and 63 percent of all psychiatrists surveyed. While differences exist, the majority of the respondents agreed that pathological gambling is very similar to drug addiction and alcoholism.

When asked if pathological gamblers usually have other severe problems in living caused by a basic character disorder rather than by an illness or addiction, only 34 percent of all GA members agreed, followed by 24 percent of all treatment experts, 35 percent of all psychologists, and 31 percent of all psychiatrists surveyed. When asked if they really don't believe there is such a thing as pathological gambling, not a single GA member agreed nor did any of the treatment experts or psychologists. Only 3 percent of all psychiatrists surveyed agreed.

The first half of Taber's survey reveals just how successful the discursive negotiations of Custer and colleagues have been over the past three decades. In fact, two of the most important of the fourteen practices Blume (1987) outlined were accepted by an overwhelmingly significant number of treatment professionals and members of Gamblers Anonymous. Most of them believed that gambling was a disease like alcoholism and drug addiction and that the problems of gambling were located in biology. The second set of questions pertain to treatment issues.

When asked if some form of professional help is necessary for pathological gamblers to permanently arrest their gambling, only 36 percent of all GA members agreed, whereas 52 percent of all treatment experts, 88 percent of all psychologists, and 72 percent of all psychiatrists agreed. This question evidences the still existing differences in discursive practice between treatment professionals and members of GA. GA members are unlikely to agree that treatment rather than GA is the cure to gambling. Unless GA is somehow involved, most GA members are suspect of medical treatment. This is an interesting set of discursive negotiations. Members of GA usually rely upon the medical model to combat public and professional ignorance and stigma about gambling, and the councils use it for the purposes of lobbying their case, and yet they disagree that, on its own, it has the power to cure pathological gambling.

This thinking reveals the complexity of discursive agency. It makes perfect sense for GA members to involve themselves in the discursive strategies of the medical model as they interact with themselves and others. But, in so doing, they negotiate these practices and modify and alter them to fit the various other practices by which they live their lives. Remember, the medical model is a negotiated order. As practiced in inter-action, members of GA are allowed to take the parts they agree with, discard the rest, and perhaps call on one set of practices in one situation while not using those same practices in another. One example is believing in the power of the medical model, but also understanding the importance of the Twelve-Steps, which is a spiritual approach to recovery.

Lastly, when asked if an alliance of professional and self-help groups working together is the ideal arrangement for helping compulsive gamblers, 74 percent of all GA members agreed, followed by 100 percent of all treatment professionals, 92 percent of all psychologists, and 91 percent of all psychiatrists surveyed. This final question clearly shows how enmeshed GA and medical treatment are. When asked if a combination of GA and medical treatment is the ideal formal discourse on gambling, the overwhelming majority are in favor.[2] The history of in-patient gambling treatment has supported this survey. It is hard to find a treatment program today that does not have some level of involvement with GA.

The National and State Councils as Discursive Political Machines

The National Council on Compulsive Gambling, as Rosecrance (1985a) explained, contains representatives from psychiatry, psychology, law, medicine, and pathological gambling. Because of its multi-disciplinary support, besides medicine and business, it has been the only other major organization with enough power to influence national discourse and affect governmental policy and public education.

As with the field of gambling treatment, the choice by the National Council to use the medical model has as much to do with authority and political power as it does with research and clinical opinion. To struggle to make changes and increase social consciousness in a political and cultural climate that is largely pro-gambling—a political and cultural climate that has chosen to ignore the heavy social consequences of gambling—the National Council has had little discursive choice. They've desperately needed a discourse powerful enough to change policy and perception. The medical model works the best because it has gotten the most accomplished when fighting for funding, education, treatment, and research. The same has been true of the various state councils and some of the national programs like the Institute for Problem Gambling and the National Center for Responsible Gaming—the first major organization to provide funding for research in gambling

Most state councils, such as the Florida Council on Compulsive Gambling and the North American Training Institute (a subdivision of the Minnesota Council on Compulsive Gambling), are aware that pathological gambling is a social issue; one that requires a discourse larger than the medical, and yet they've been in a tough situation. If they are to negotiate with business and government, they've got to refrain from being too critical. Sociology is critical and often alienates business. Plus, most councils have been so busy helping communities already struggling with gambling, that they've had little time to do the research and investigation necessary to call attention to the larger social problem. As a result, the councils have found themselves in a catch-22: if they don't use the medical model, they lose their power and position, but by using the medical model they lack the discursive power necessary to call attention to the larger social problems—such as the excessive gambling of the elderly. And so, they've done what they can, while hoping for further research to make the larger social issues known. To date, these more sociological articles have not been written.

Benefiting from the Medical Model

The list of benefits GA receives from the medical model are many (e.g., respect, authority, and public attention). One of the most important is overcoming the legal and moral stigma historically attached to pathological gambling. As Rose (1988) and others in the sociology of deviance have pointed out (e.g., Conrad and Schneider 1980), it is far better for an individual living in the 1990s to blame their problems on a disease than to be given responsibility because they have sinned or because they lack the will-power. The disease concept frees people from their past. Members of GA can gain understanding, compassion, and tolerance if people understand they suffer from a disease. The medical model challenges people—from judges and police officers to family members and casinos—to change their opinions about the excesses and problems of gambling. You cannot blame a person for being sick. You can be angry with their past behaviors, but you cannot ostracize them for having an illness.

The second most important benefit is freedom from a certain amount of responsibility for past actions. Clients often say: I was different before I started gambling. When I was younger I was honest, caring, a good husband, a productive worker. I never lied. I never stole a thing. I can't stand myself now. I can't believe I did the things I did. I had to be insane. Therapists respond: You need to stop beating yourself up so much. If you cannot get past the guilt, you are never going to recover. You need to make amends with the past and move on. These therapists have a point. I have worked with clients unable to get past their guilt and self-hate. They are their own worst enemy. I challenged them to accept and learn from their past mistakes, forgive themselves, and then move on—otherwise they remain within a world of psychological and emotional despair that damages those around them as much as themselves.

If you notice, my treatment recommendation has nothing to do with relieving responsibility. Quite the opposite, the person embraces past mistakes, learns from them, and heals. The medical model—even when used by therapists who embrace the complex issues of rehabilitation and responsibility—however, does not always foster this type of behavior. It tends to externalize pathological gambling as if it were a foreign agent or host. Patient—if they so desire and often enough do—can easily use this discourse to manipulate others.

The tendency of patients to use the medical model to their advantage has been recently documented in a study by Wedgeworth (1998). Wedgeworth found that most people coming in for gambling treatment do so because they wish to resolve some type of gambling related crisis in their lives—be it a problem with a family member, a boss, or the court. Most pathological gamblers, in order to gamble, often get their money from a small network of people. They've relied on these people to take care of them, give them money, bail them out. These people are the co-dependents. Often, it is only when these gamblers have brought one or more of these various relationships to the verge of total destruction that they seek treatment. They use treatment, therapists, the clinic, the diagnosis, and the medical model to get themselves out of this trouble. They lean up against, manipulate, and distort all of these various people and discourses to obtain their goal: the re-connection and re-establishment of one or more of their relations. Sometimes it works, sometimes it doesn't. Again, this process does not describe all patients, but everyone—all of us—uses knowledge at some level to deal with the tough issue of responsibility.

The third and most important benefit GA and the Council gain from adhering to the medical model is the benefit of treatment. In our hyper-medicalized, individualistic, capitalistic, non-sociologically thinking society, unless there is a professionally recognized medical diagnosis for a social problem, third-party payment cannot be collected. Even though pathological gambling was included in 1980 in the DSM-III, insurance companies, even today, are only beginning to recognize pathological gambling as a treatable diagnosis for which they need to provide payment. If the Councils and GA are to get anywhere, they've got to use the medical model. Goodman (1995) explains: "In the past, most health insurance companies tended to view compulsive gambling as a moral problem, a lack of responsible behavior rather than a disease, and would not pay for treatment of problem gamblers. But as the problem increased, and counselors became more sophisticated in dealing with insurance companies, treatment payments began to be more readily available. In some cases, according to a 1992 report in the *New York Times,* treatment centers find ways to call gambling problems "depression"—a medical condition that insurance companies will cover" (p. 54). And so we have the reasons why the medical model has been so enticing.

GA and the National and State Gambling Councils as Discursive Foot Soldiers

While GA and the Councils have certainly benefited from the medical model, so has the medical model benefited from them. For example, without the support of GA, Custer never would have come to the realization that pathological gambling required treatment. It was also through GA that the disease concept of gambling gained public support and attention. As more and more of the middle-classes began attending GA meetings, they became educated in the GA hybrid of the medical discourse. They then carried these perceptions with them as they sought out professional treatment.

The National Council on Problem Gambling, like the AMA (American Medical Association), has been the primary liaison between medical researchers and treatment centers and the general public. By organizing research and publishing it to circulate to a readership that goes beyond the professional audience to policy makers and other philanthropists, the Council has clearly charted the medical model's future. As the Council made its position known during the 1980s and 1990s, its web of discursive relations spread outward, affecting state politicians, government, the gambling industry, churches, and so on. Thus, the Council's discursive negotiations over the past twenty years have acted like outward ripples in a pool, leaving their impact felt across the entire country. As we turn to the next century, these ripples will probably become more like waves.

usage of psychiatric knowledge. Others wanted to ban the insanity defense altogether. Dr. Halpern was one of these psychiatrists. He was renown for his objection to the insanity defense.

During the early 1980s, in reaction to the rising concerns Halpern and others raised concerning the insanity defense, the American Psychiatric Association put together a group of leading experts in forensic psychiatry to publish a formal statement on the insanity defense which would represent the views of mainstream American psychiatry. They called the group the Insanity Defense Work Group. The title of the article, which was published in 1983, the same year as Torniero's case, was the "American Psychiatric Association Statement on the Insanity Defense." The committee came out in favor of the insanity defense, but offered a number of important caveats to the usage of psychiatric knowledge and provided several useful suggestions for the criminal justice system to consider. Two of the key members of this committee were Alan A. Stone, M.D. and Robert Spitzer, M.D. During his testimony, Halpern talked about his interactions with Dr. Stone over the construction of the American Psychiatric Association's statement on the insanity defense. He even read a letter addressed to him from Dr. Stone where Stone questioned Halpern's virulence toward the committee's final decision.[1] According to Halpern, Dr. Stone and the rest of the committee neither sought out nor included his opinions about the insanity defense, which he believed a significant number of people within psychiatry shared with him. Nevertheless, Halpern used the Torniero case as a forum to express and discursively negotiate his views, hoping that what he had to say would affect the future of the insanity defense within the Federal Court, Second Circuit. Hartmere supported Halpern's agenda.

Having used Dr. Halpern's testimony to make the wider claim that the insanity defense itself was worthy of question, Hartmere settled in to take apart the defense's argument. Two issues were at stake if Hartmere was to prove the defense wrong. First, he needed to throw into question the validity of the DSM-III diagnosis of pathological gambling itself by focusing in on a distinction between two phrases "unable to resist the impulse to gamble" versus "failure to resist the impulse to gamble." The second and final agenda of Hartmere was to make the distinction between the clinical and legal definition of insanity. If Hartmere could prove that the clinical definition of insanity is different from the legal, and that the clinical definition is inappropriate in a court of law, then he could argue that, despite the severity of pathological gambling, it was not an appropriate defense of insanity. Hartmere's star witness was Dr. Stephen Rachlin.

At the time of the trial, Dr. Rachlin, a forensic psychiatrist by training, had neither treated nor done research on pathological gambling; in fact, he wasn't even current on the pathological gambling literature—other than what the prosecution had presented to him in their Brandeis-brief and a few outside articles. This didn't matter though, because his importance to the trial was found elsewhere in his credentials. As a forensic psychiatrist he was a leading expert on the insanity defense and, most importantly, a colleague of Dr. Halpern. While a colleague of Halpern's, Rachlin, surprisingly, was not opposed to the continued usage of the insanity defense and was in agreement with the American Psychiatric Association's published article on the insanity defense—which surprisingly ran counter to Hartmere's larger agenda. Rachlin's support of the insanity defense came out during Keefe's cross-examination:

BY MR. KEEFE:

Q Well, [Dr. Rachlin] are you in favor of retention of the insanity defense?

A Yes, . . .

Q And so you do not agree with Dr. Halpern's position that it out to be abolished in toto?

A I do not agree with that position.

Q And, in fact, I think you told Mr. Hartmere a few minutes ago that you are in agreement with the APA recommendation as to their insanity defense proposal which is contained in the document before you, Government Exhibit 8, is that correct?

A That is correct. It recommends narrowing in two specific directions.

Q All right. And with those amendments, sir, or proposed amendments, you are in favor of retention of the insanity defense as proposed by the American Psychiatric Association?

A Yes, I think my own personal position is tremendously in congruence with the American Psychiatric Association's position. (United States vs. John J. Torniero, 1983 Criminal 82–1106, pp. 201–202)

While not opposed to the insanity defense as a whole, Rachlin was, most importantly, opposed to the further usage of pathological gambling as the basis for such a defense. It was for this reason that Hartmere called him to the witness stand:

BY MR. HARTMERE:

Q Now, going back, Doctor, based on your research and your interest in pathological gambling, what is your opinion as to the use of pathological gambling as an insanity defense in a criminal prosecution?

A My opinion literally over the past 15 years is that the diagnosis of pathological gambling or compulsive gambling, with no other psychiatric diagnosis, should in no way lead to consideration of an insanity defense.

Q Now, why do you believe that?

A I believe that for several reasons, one of which is that it is, as we said a moment ago, to repeat, partly defined by the criminal behavior that it's then thought to be used as exculpatory.

I believe that because I see the entity of pathological gambling as being both qualitatively and quantitatively different from the serious mental illnesses which do, in fact, qualify for an insanity defense. (United States vs. John J. Torniero, 1983 Criminal 82–1106, p. 195)

With Dr. Rachlin, Hartmere had one of his star witnesses: a psychiatrist in direct opposition to the testimonies of Custer and Taber. At the time of the above questioning, Hartmere was trying to reveal the duality of the diagnosis of pathological gambling. One of the primary problems with the DSM is that it defines pathological gambling, in part, by its criminal behavior. In the *DSM-III,* for example, two of the key symptoms are

a) arrest for forgery, fraud, embezzlement, or income tax evasion due to attempts to obtain money for gambling, and b) borrowing of money from illegal sources (American Psychiatric Association 1980, p. 291). If criminal behavior revolving around finances is one of *the* key defining features of pathological gambling, then it is not only a clinical problem. It has aspects of both the criminal and the clinical. It is this very issue that makes pathological gambling such a difficult issue to resolve. It is as much a criminal problem as it is a medical one. Hartmere wanted to show that it is more criminal than clinical. He continued to strengthen his argument by asking Rachlin to compare pathological gambling to other major disorders. First Hartmere asked Rachlin if pathological gambling was a psychosis. Rachlin said "No." Later in his questioning he asked if pathological gambling was a neurosis. Again, Rachlin said "No, I would not so categorize it." Like Custer and the others, Rachlin provided clinical cases to support his position.

Having adequately put into question the severity of pathological gambling, Hartmere next focused in on the wording of the DSM-III itself. This was to be his primary point of attack. The point of contention Hartmere and others had with the DSM-III—and the reason is was radically changed for the DSM-III-R—was the opening statement of the diagnostic table. It stated: "The individual is chronically and progressively *unable* to resist impulses to gamble" (American Psychiatric Association 1980, p. 292, italics mine). What had made other defenses of insanity so successful following the DSM-III publication was the word *unable*. If someone is *unable* to resist the impulse to gamble, then they are not in control of their behavior. They are insane enough to have lost rational control. If being *out of control* for pathological gamblers is defined, in part, by criminal activity, then their criminal behavior is, by definition, a function of their insanity. Hartmere had to prove this wrong. His argument to prove the DSM-III wrong was that pathological gamblers are not *unable to resist* the impulse to gamble, they *fail to resist* the impulse. The way he tried to prove the defense wrong was by focusing on the opening line of the diagnosis itself. While the diagnosis table used the word *unable*, the opening line of the diagnosis itself used the word *failure*:

> 312.31 Pathological Gambling.
>
> The essential features are a chronic and progressive *failure* to resist impulses to gambling and gambling behavior that

compromises, disrupts, or damages personal, family, or vocational pursuits." (DSM-III, 1980, p. 291, italics mine)

If Hartmere could convince the judge that the opening line of the diagnosis was more important than the opening line of the table itself, then he would win his argument. Hartmere started his line of questioning with Dr. Rachlin:

BY MR. HARTMERE

Q Now, [Dr. Rachlin] have you reviewed Government Exhibit 6, which are the appendixes to Part IV of the Government's motion to reconsider the law of insanity?

A Yes, I read the testimony at that trial transcript.

Q And specifically did you read the testimony of Dr. Ames Robey in that case?

A Yes, I did specifically read his testimony.

Q And do you agree with what Dr. Robey testified to?

A I agree fully with Dr. Robey.

Q And who is Dr. Robey?

A Dr. Robey is a forensic psychiatrist of many years' experience, and at least a national reputation, who practices currently in Michigan, and for a while was Medical Director of their Center For Forensic Psychiatry.

Q And do you know what his conclusion was in the case in the Southern District of Iowa in his testimony?

A His essential conclusion was that the disorder of pathological gambling did not rise to the level of mental disease or defect in the sense that it was used in the ALI test of non-responsibility. (United States vs. John J. Torniero, 1983 Criminal 82–1106, pp. 196–197)

While Dr. Robey was not a witness at the Torniero trial, his opinions on the issue of pathological gambling were highly important and included in Hartmere's Appellate Court Brief. They delivered a devastating blow to the defense's arguments. At the time of the trial, Dr. Ames Robey was a leading forensic psychiatrist and founding member of the American Academy of Psychiatry and Law. Robey had been "instrumental in drafting the language used to describe pathological gambling in the DSM-III."[2] In a similar trial (United States vs. Lewellyn 1983), Dr. Robey testified that when the diagnosis of pathological gambling was constructed, it was written with the specific attempt to keep it outside the domain of the legal definition of insanity. The confusion that emerged out of the contradiction between the words *unable* and *failure* was a huge mistake on their part, and that if either of the two words were to be favored, it would be the word *failure*. The following comes from Dr. Robey's testimony at the Lewellyn trial:

> [A]ny lack of substantial capacity to conform one's behavior to the requirements of the law must be . . . 'by reason of mental disease or defect.' And it was in this area that not only Dr. Spitzer in the APA group, but also our advisory group, were very clear to list this as a separate group: . . . "impulse disorders not elsewhere classified." And by definition the impulse disorder is not a mental defect. And it is primarily for this reason . . . that it fails to meet the test, and was designed to fail to meet the test for that reason.
>
> Further, however, the inability to conform, the lack of substantial capacity to be able to conform one's behavior to the requirements of the law, is broken down, in the case of the compulsive gambler, into gambling, which is and of itself, at least in many jurisdictions, is not exactly illegal, although it's sometimes extra-legal, but goes much more to the separate issue of his subsequent actions in terms of having to recoup his losses. And the inability to avoid forgery, tax evasion, embezzlement is clearly there, and the extent, indeed, to which these individuals go to carefully conceal their sources of money, to be able to continue it, is far more socio-pathic, far more antisocial, and doesn't come anywhere close to falling into anything mentally ill. It is an offshoot of their gambling, and even if one wished to consider that an illness, the embezzlement or criminal activities that arise from it are clearly unresisted impulses, not the

> result of any insufficient capability to conform their behavior to the requirements of the law. (United States of America v. John Torniero, 1983 No. 83–1459, Brief for the Appellee, pp. 8–9. United States Court of Appeals for the Second Circuit)

There it was. The writers of the diagnosis itself, based on their psychiatric expertise, never intended the diagnosis to be used as the basis for an insanity defense. Hartmere had his first argument accomplished. The DSM-III itself, as far as its wording was concerned, could not be trusted beyond its usage in a clinical setting. It was faulty. During the pre-trial hearing itself, Hartmere made the same argument using the testimony of Dr. Halpern.

Although Dr. Halpern was Hartmere's star witness on the issue of the insanity defense as a whole, Halpern—who had never done therapy or research with pathological gamblers—had a strong opinion on the wording of the DSM-III. Halpern had taken it upon himself to check any and all new diagnoses added to each publication of the DSM. Whenever he found a diagnosis which he felt was not appropriate for a defense of insanity, he would check the diagnosis for potential legal misrepresentation. When he saw the contradiction between the words *failure* and *inability,* he wrote Dr. Spitzer, one of the members of the Insanity Defense Work Group and a part of the DSM revision committee, to suggest the words be changed. Hartmere brought the correspondence between Halpern and Spitzer during his questioning of Halpern.

> BY MR. HARTMERE:
>
> Q Doctor [Halpern,] I am placing before you Government 13 and 14 for identification. Do you recognize those two documents, two letters?
>
> A Yes sir.
>
> Q And what are they? Without reading them, just what do they deal with?
>
> A Well, this is an exchange of communications between myself and Dr. Robert Spitzer, the developer and chief author of the DSM-III. . . .
>
> Q Doctor, would you just read Government 13, please?

A Read it sir?

Q Yes, please.

A All right. This is a letter on my letterhead dated July 23, 1980 to Robert L. Spitzer, MD, Chief of Psychiatric Research, Biometrics Research Department, New York State Psychiatric Institute . . .

"Dear Bob: The first sentence under DSM-III 312.31 (pathological gambling) properly includes the words 'failure to resist impulses to gamble,' whereas, unfortunately, the 'diagnostic criteria for pathological gambling' on page 292 uses the expression 'unable to resist impulses to gamble.' "

"I strongly recommend that criterion A in the next edition of DSM-III be corrected to read as follows: 'The individual chronically and progressively fails to resist impulses to gamble. . . .' "

"Best Regards, Sincerely."

Q Okay. And did you receive a response from Dr. Spitzer?

A I received a response from Dr. Spitzer dated August 5, 1980, addressed to me and reading as follows:

"Dear Abe: Thank you for your July 23rd letter. It makes a lot of sense and we will propose it for the next revision of DSM-III."

"Sincerely yours, Robert L. Spitzer, MD, Chief of Psychiatric Research, Biometrics Research Department." (United States vs. John J. Torniero, 1983 Criminal 82–1106, pp. 170–171)

Again, Hartmere had accomplished his task. The creators of the DSM itself admitted, in letter, that the diagnosis of pathological gambling was legally problematic in its wording. It needed to be changed. While it should be taken into consideration for purposes of punishment and treatment, it is not a diagnosis appropriate for the defense of insanity.

In his cross-examination, Keefe tried to refute Hartmere's argument. The leading experts testified that pathological gamblers, in the desperation phase, are unable to resist impulses to gamble. That's why the word *unable* is in the table. Besides, Hartmere's witnesses, both Halpern and

Rachlin, had never treated or done research on pathological gambling. How would they know? Their arguments were based on discourse alone, not experience. Real live experience. Keefe went after Rachlin on this point, but Rachlin stuck to his story. Pathological gamblers *are* able to control their impulses, they simply *fail* to do so.

BY MR. KEEFE

Q Well, sir, under the diagnostic criteria for pathological gambling, that heading, it says that the defendant must be chronically and progressively unable to resist the impulse to gamble; correct?

A That's what it says.

Q All right. And that heading lists, as it says, the diagnostic criteria for pathological gambling, right?

A Correct.

Q And nowhere else in this entire bible [Keefe is referring to the DSM-III] does it list the diagnostic criteria for pathological gambling?

A That's correct.

Q And when someone is unable chronically, that means permanently, doesn't it, or long term?

A Long term.

Q And progressively, that means increasingly so; correct?

A Yes.

Q And when someone is chronically, or long term, and progressively, increasingly, unable to resist an impulse, that person is really mentally ill, isn't he?

A Maybe.

Q Well, isn't he always if he can't resist, if he's unable to resist an impulse?

A I would not use that one criteria alone to diagnose mental illness, no, not on the basis of that one criteria alone.

Q In other words, in your opinion, if a person is long term unable to resist an impulse and it's getting worse, it's getting progressively worse, that alone, no matter what the impulse is, does not qualify for mental illness?

A I need to know more about it, yes. . . .

Q All right. And I take it you agree with that definition of pathological gambling?

A Yes, that—well, I do not agree with the term "unable." I have that quibble with the definition, yes. Otherwise, no problem.

Q So as I understand it, you would delete the term "unable" and substitute what—"unwilling?"

A Failure to resist impulses, as on page 291 in the discussion of this condition.

Q All right. But that's a discussion, that's not listing the diagnostic criteria, is it?

A You're correct.

Q All right. So you would change it to even make pathological gambling, sir, the standard to be a pathological gambler, you would lessen the standards, is that right?

A In the sense of making "unable to" "failure to," yes. (United States vs. John J. Torniero, 1983 Criminal 82–1106, pp. 227–230)

With his first major argument complete, Hartmere next focused on the difference between the clinical and legal definitions of insanity. The problem between a legal and clinical conception of insanity has to do with the different purposes and uses of the term *mental disease*. Insanity is a legal term. It is not used in treatment. In treatment, the term insanity is viewed as pejorative. Treatment professionals use the term *mental disease* or *mental disorder* to refer to those problems that traditionally fall within the realm of insanity. A mental disorder, according to the DSM-III, "is conceptualized as a clinically significant behavioral or psychological syndrome or pattern that occurs in an individual and that is typically associated with either a painful symptom (distress) or impairment in one or more important areas of functioning (disability). In addition, there is an inference that there is a behavioral, psychological, or biological dysfunction, and that the disturbance is not only in the relationship between the individual and society. (When the disturbance is limited to a conflict between an individual and society, this may represent social deviance, which may or may not be commendable, but is not by itself a mental disorder.)" (American Psychiatric Association 1980, p. 6). In contrast, the criminal justice system uses the term *mental disorder* or *mental illness* to explain why certain defendants lack the ability to distinguish between right and wrong, or lack an appreciation for what they are doing. In short, the criminal justice system uses the term mental disorder strictly for the purposes of distinguishing between defendants who are and are not responsible for their behavior. Nothing else. As noted gambling law professor Rose (1988) stated, when it comes to criminal insanity, "[t]he particular defendant is either acting out of free will and is therefore liable for his actions, or is ill and cannot be held responsible. Guilty or innocent" (p. 257). One way or the other, a decision must be made. In the clinical realm no such distinction is necessary. In fact, issues of responsibility are irrelevant. The diagnosis of mental disorder exists to help clinicians understand common problems in a manner that allows them to talk with one another and provide effective treatment. In the case of pathological gambling, the words *unable* and *failure* are used to give a certain clinical impression. They are not used to make distinctions in the case of legal responsibility. As soon as issues of responsibility emerge, the law must be present. Bottom line, Hartmere's argument is that while pathological gambling was codified as a mental disorder in the DSM, it was never intended to be used in a legal context. Therefore, any reference to pathological gambling as a mental illness or disorder by psychiatry, psychology or medicine is strictly for clinical purposes only. When it comes to pathological gambling, no defense should misrepresent the terms *mental disorder* by attempting to reframe it as the legal basis for a defense of insanity. Hartmere made his point clear in his redirect examination with Dr. Rachlin.

BY MR. HARTMERE:

Q Doctor, did you just testify, in response to Mr. Keefe, that for clinical purposes mental disorder is a mental disease, in your opinion?

A Yes.

Q What did you mean by "for clinical purposes?"

A In terms of classification, treatment, planning, those are, to me, the two critical issues: diagnosis and treatment.
Patient care in its broadest sense is what I mean by "clinical."

Q Is that different than mental disease in terms of a court of law? Is there a distinction between for clinical purposes and for legal purposes?

A Yes, absolutely.

Q And what is the distinction, in your opinion?

A Well, for example, in the ALI test of insanity it speaks of mental disease or defect, and all disorders to rise to the level of disease or defects. They may be disorders for our treatment or evaluation purposes, they need not necessarily be diseases for legal purposes. . . .

Q Now, do you consider yourself an expert in psychiatry?

A Yes, I do.

Q And an expert in forensic psychiatry?

A Yes, I do.

Q Is it fair to say that there are hundreds of disorders, mental disorders?

A Yes.

Q Are you an expert in each one of those disorders?

A No, not necessarily in each individual one.

Q Do you know anyone who is?

A No.

Q And what is the purpose of the DSM-III?

A Its purpose, if I can go back to my definition of "clinical," its purpose is for clinical uses. It is designed to achieve agreement on diagnostic classification for the purposes of formulating appropriate treatment for individuals with each of these conditions. Obviously, the treatment of all these hundreds of conditions is as different as the conditions themselves are.

Q Is it fair to say that it's a diagnostic and treatment manual?

A It is a diagnostic manual from which treatment will flow. . . .

Q Is DSM-III a forensic manual?

A No, it is not specifically a forensic manual.

Q And, in fact, on directing your attention to page 12 of your DSM-III, is there a caution that appears on page 12?

A There is a caution listed.

Q Would you read it?

A Shall I read it?

Q Yes, please.

A "The purpose of the DSM-III is to provide clear descriptions of diagnostic categories in order to enable clinicians and investigators to diagnose, communicate about, study and treat various mental disorders. The use of this manual for non-clinical purposes, such as determination of legal responsibility, competency or insanity, or justification for third party payments, must be critically examined in each instance within the appropriate institutional context."

Mr. Hartmere: Thank you, Dr. Rachlin. I have nothing further, your Honor. (United States vs. John J. Torniero, 1983 Criminal 82–1106, pp. 245–249)

With his second and final point made, Hartmere finished the presentation of his argument, the rest was cross-examining Keefe's witnesses and re-examining his own. Hartmere's concluding remarks about the case were published in his Appellee Brief: "The Government suggests that by definition, pathological gambling is not a serious mental illness, and therefore not a mental disease or defect contemplated in the ALI test of criminal responsibility."[3]

Chapter 8

THE GAMBLING INDUSTRY

While neither state level government nor the gambling industry were called as witnesses on behalf of the prosecution, during the 1980s and 1990s they certainly were the two biggest supporters of the arguments put forth by Hartmere.

What is interesting about the government and the gambling industry is that, despite their differences, for the past eighteen years they've basically remained true to the belief that gambling is primarily a harmless, rational activity that the overwhelming majority (97 percent of the population) participate in with little to no consequences. While some people gamble to excess, it is largely a function of their own pathology, not the gambling itself. These people should receive treatment if necessary, but government and business shouldn't be blamed for these problems, and neither should they be held responsible for the financial debts and legal consequences incurred by individuals otherwise labeled as "pathological gamblers." Regardless of their pathology, if someone has committed a crime or owes someone else money (particularly a casino), they must be held responsible to the requirements of the law just like anybody else.

Given the similarities between government and the gambling industry, three questions immediately emerge. First of all, how and why did these two different forces come to the same basic conclusion that the medical model of pathological gambling is of little concern to the general population? Did they reach these conclusions as a function of research and clinical investigation alone or were socio-historical, political, institutional, professional, and economic factors involved as well? Second, how exactly did they marginalize the medical model? Did they just ignore it or did they lobby against it? And third, what were the consequences of their response to the medical model? How have their arguments affected the people who struggle with this disorder? To answer these questions, we start with the gambling industry.

Is Gambling Pathological?
Comments from the Gambling Industry

In 1993 and 1994, Nicholas A. Spano, a pro-gambling senator from New York, put together a subcommittee to determine if casinos could be built in the Catskills. The committee's goal was to conduct an objective and unbiased examination into the issue. "But," writes Goodman (1995), "a close reading of the subcommittee's report makes clear that those who presented information that argued against legalization were summarily dismissed as biased, while those who favored legalized gambling were accorded a cordial and receptive hearing" (p. 67). In fact, the subcommittee dismissed a report submitted by Howard Shaffer, Director of the Center for Addiction Studies at Harvard Medical School, as biased because "it was prepared for the Massachusetts Council on Compulsive Gambling, whose funding, the subcommittee complained, 'is derived from showing that problem or pathological gambling is a serious problem'" (p. 68). Meanwhile, "the subcommittee had no difficulty accepting at face value a number of unsubstantiated and clearly absurd statements by gambling industry representatives" (p. 68). One such statement came from Paul Dorwin, the publisher and editor of *Gaming & Wagering Business,* who reported that, according to his sources, people only go to casinos for entertainment: "they do not go because they have or want to win money" (p. 68). During the meeting, the subcommittee also heard reports from three of the top gambling industry corporations, Caesar's World, Hilton, and Promus (Harrah's Casinos). The representatives for these hotels were quoted as "experts" on the problems of gambling and extensively cited throughout the report.

Given its pro-gambling position, the gambling industry during the 1980s and 1990s became increasingly concerned with the problems of pathological gambling, but not necessarily because they wanted to fix them. They had other motives—primarily two. First, people with gambling problems don't pay back their debts (e.g., Barton 1990; Kennedy 1994; Lewis 1986; Zorn 1995). Second, gambling casinos, in the advent of the disease model of gambling, are liable for law suits (e.g., Wolfe 1995). Rose (1988) explains:

> The growing conflict in the law over how to deal with compulsive gambling is coming to a head in cases involving legal gambling. The legal gambling industry would suffer a terrible financial blow if this doctrine [—that compulsive gamblers suffer from a disease and are therefore insane and not legally responsible for their criminal actions or gambling debts—] were generally accepted. Their immediate concern are cases in which the gambler argues that he is not liable for his gambling debts because he is a compulsive gambler. Casinos in particular rely upon liberal credit policies; if any player could raise compulsive gambling as a possible defense, collection of small debts would become extremely expensive and many large debts would be uncollectable. However, every form of gambling, from racetracks, through state lotteries, to stock brokers would be open to suits whenever anyone lost money. . . . (Pp. 253–254)

While their motives are economically driven, the argument raised by the gambling industry is important. Are not diagnosed pathological gamblers required to account for their actions in a court of law? Are not these people responsible to make amends to their families, their friends, employers, loan agencies, bookies, and so on? As citizens, regardless of sickness or disease, can these people be excused from their social contract? It was these types of questions that one of the gambling industry's own attempted to answer: attorney, Shannon Bybee.

A View from the Gambling Industry: Shannon Bybee and Problem Gambling

Of the various formal discourses available on the issue of the excesses and problems of gambling, an example of the general position taken by the gambling industry comes from Shannon Bybee's 1988 article, "Problem

Gambling: One View from the Gambling Industry Side." It was published in Rose and Lorenz's special edited issue "Compulsive Gambling And The Law," (1988) for *The Journal Of Gambling Behavior.* Rose and Lorenz's special edition was the first and only major collection of inter-disciplinary writings on the issue of compulsive gambling and the law.

At the time of the article, Bybee held a major position in the gambling industry. He was a licensed attorney and consultant in Las Vegas, Nevada. During his career he was also a regulator of the gaming industry in Nevada, president of a casino hotel in New Jersey, a legal representative for several casino operators in Nevada, and a lobbyist for casinos in New Jersey (Bybee 1988, p. 302).

The argument Bybee made in his 1988 article was similar to arguments being made by the gambling industry at the time. The gambling industry is, for the most part, a benign business institution, no different in its operation than, say, K-Mart. The goal is to make a profit. It makes a profit by providing people the opportunity to gamble. It does not go out and drag people in. People transport themselves to casinos, race tracks, and river boats because they want to gamble. It is as simple as that. Gambling is a rational behavior, a leisure activity, a social past-time which has finally lost the moral overtones that past generations held over it. The gambling industry is another advancement in democratic freedom. United States society has always liked to gamble. Now they can. If poor people spend their income on gambling, is it the gambling industry's fault? Is the industry responsible for monitoring people's checkbooks? Should they stop advertising just because a small minority of people don't know how to control themselves? Why should the gambling industry be held to higher standards than other businesses? Why is it that the gambling industry should be responsible for providing financial aid for education, research, and treatment? Why should they support a medical model of treatment? Why should they not be allowed to make a profit as other companies do? What other businesses are called to be so socially and clinically responsible? Does Coca-Cola provide monies for the potential of caffeine addiction? Bybee (1988) clarified this position even more:

> There has been considerable effort by some to view problem gambling as an isolated problem. This makes shifting the blame from the individual to the casino much easier and much neater. It also makes industry funding sound almost reasonable. But

> the pigeonhole approach to funding and fault-shifting in this area is an inadequate and unfair approach to a problem that just does not fit into pigeonholes.
>
> Problem gamblers are seldom people whose only aberrant behavior is over-indulgence in gambling. They often overindulge in other areas as well. The issue of "poly-addiction" is being increasingly recognized along with the recognition that treatment should address all aspects of "compulsive" behavior exhibited by a person. An individual who manifests multiple forms of the problem should not have to go to multiple locations and receive similar treatments from multiple professionals. Cause and effect become difficult to assess, as well as financial responsibility for treatment and study, when we deal with all aspects of this type of behavior and separate them into pigeonholes. Those whose only concern is alcoholism or drug abuse or problem gambling would prefer to keep it in separate pigeonholes. Sometimes professionals whose expertise is in one of these areas have an ego, and perhaps even financial, interest in maintaining the pigeonhole approach to the problem.
>
> Instead of trying to pry money out of the gaming industry or any other industry on the basis of fault-shifting, there should be greater emphasis on combining resources to deal with these various types of destructive behaviors and funding should come from a broad base, because it really is a broad base problem—not just a gaming industry problem. (Pp. 305–306)

A number of interpretations can be made from Bybee's quote. First, note the contradictions in Bybee's logic. He purports that the entire argument put forth by the medical model is based on economic incentive and the desire to maintain professional authority and power. But, how are the goals of the gambling industry any different? In order to manipulate the consumer, and to sway moral and cultural opinion to the side of pro-gambling, the industry engages in the same type of discursive negotiations. Within the past several years, the gambling industry has changed its name from the *gambling industry* to the *gaming industry.* Likewise, Las Vegas is no longer a gambling town. The casinos have spent millions and millions of dollars to change their image. They've removed all of the prostitutes from the main drag; they've cleaned up their streets, and started advertizing themselves as a "family vacation" hot spot. In fact, Las Vegas is currently the second fastest growing city in the United States, it has one of the lowest crime rates in the country. The gambling industry also makes contributions to charities and, sometimes, provides money for research, education, and treatment. All of this is done for one reason: to protect the image of the gambling industry for the purposes of making money. Even in his article, Bybee plays a game of words. If you spend some time looking at Bybee's article, you see that he uses the term *problem gambler* instead of *pathological gambler, over-indulgence* instead of *compulsion* or *addiction,* and *aberrant behavior* instead of *disease.* Bybee's choice of vocabulary is a specific attempt to avoid the language of medicine and psychology. As a result, Bybee's argument is just as potentially problematic as the discourse he is attacking.

Bybee's concerns with the medical model do not stop with gambling treatment alone. He believes that the United States as a whole has been seduced into the *disease model* of addiction. He (1988) states:

> In the past year television news and talk shows have featured people with such "problem" activities as "compulsive" shopping and sex. There is more evidence each year that many people have a problem resisting impulses to engage in some activity to the point of causing problems for themselves and others. Problem gamblers are not unique, and neither is the gaming industry when it comes to this issue.
>
> But, as Professor I. Nelson Rose observed, there is increasing acceptance for the assumption that a gambler who gambles to excess "is an individual who suffers from a disease and is thus not responsible for his actions." This is part of a greater movement that has attempted to make society or corporations or government responsible for everything negative and relieve individuals of responsibility. Under this view, individuals only have rights, not responsibilities; responsibility is a collective thing. This school of thought has had increasing success in making the label "compulsive gambler" stick, thus conveying the impression that the person who gambles to excess is a victim. And if there is a victim, there must be a guilty party—the casino, the racetrack or the lottery. (P. 303)

Bybee argues that the primary problem with the medical model is that it is used by pathological gamblers to escape responsibility for their actions. Instead of doing what is "right" and holding these people accountable, the field of gambling treatment and the self-help groups, because of personal, professional, institutional and economic motivation, supports them. The gaming industry cannot continue to stand by and be blamed for something it is no more responsible for than anyone or anything else.

According to Bybee, the medical model allows pathological gamblers to escape responsibility because of the mixed message it sends. On one hand, the individual is excused of all past behavior, and yet the success of treatment is based on taking responsibility in the future. Bybee (1988) states: "[R]ead what a treatment center says in a piece written to inform gamblers and their families about the treatment for problem gambling:

> It is our view that pathological gambling is a disorder or illness primarily because the victim cannot arrest the gambling behavior without intervention; that is, he cannot stop without help from others. . . . In addition, it is our view that gambling is an illness in the sense that *it is not the gambler's fault* that he or she has lost control of gambling. Blame and guilt are useless and interfere with progress. (P. 304)

After quoting from the above pamphlet, Bybee (1988) goes on to point out that the pamphlet comes from one of the leading treatment programs in the United States, "The Brecksville Program for the Treatment of Compulsive Gambling, Brecksville Division, Cleveland Veterans Administration Medical Center" (p. 304). Bybee continues: "After telling the problem gambler that he is 'sick,' through no fault of his own, the Brecksville people go on to say that gambling is *not* a sickness in the sense than a sickness can be 'cured' by someone with special healing techniques. In their view, pathological gambling is never really eliminated but can only be controlled so that it is no longer a disability" (p. 304). Again, he quotes from the pamphlet:

> The victim must be willing to do most of the actual work. The professional is, at best, a teacher and advisor; no one can as-

> sume responsibility for anyone else's gambling. So, although we believe that the gambler has an illness that is out of control, we do not treat the problem with traditional medical methods. The gambler is expected to become fully responsible for this treatment and his life in general. (P. 304)

Bybee feels that the Brecksville treatment brochure demonstrates what he calls an *Alice in Wonderland* approach to the problem of excessive gambling. Treatment professionals, in their attempt to help clients, use words such as *illness* and *disease* to mean anything they wish them to mean. Just like the Mad Hatter in *Alice,* gambling experts speak but make no sense; that is, until their discourse is put into the appropriate context. He (1988) states:

> The writer of the Brecksville pamphlet notes, quite accurately: "In treating gambling as a mental disorder we gain many significant advantages; the classification of compulsive gambling as a mental illness has important psychological, social, legal, and financial consequences." And the consequences are not just for the person with the problem. The psychological, social, legal, and financial consequences for problem gambling researchers and treatment professionals should not be underestimated as a motivating factor in their defending and maintaining the "medical" model. (P. 305)

And so, for Bybee, the medical model is a contradiction in terms constructed solely for the political, social, institutional, professional, legal, cultural, and personal benefits it provides. "I am appalled," writes Bybee, "that people claiming a science background can, without embarrassment, take the position that a person has an 'uncontrollable' impulse to gamble, or is 'addicted' to gambling, or is 'compelled' to gamble, and is therefore not responsible for having a gambling problem, but can only be helped if he has the desire to be helped, if he makes a decision to overcome the problem, and if he takes responsibility for his life" (p. 305).

Bybee believes that there are two important negative consequences that emerge from the medicalization of pathological gambling. First, because emphasis is put on the gambling industry, government escapes blame. If responsibility is going to be turned away from the problem gambler onto the social, then responsibility should be evenly distributed: "Governmental support for studies and treatment should be encouraged. The benefits and problems associated with gamblers are broad based and the associated costs should be spread over the same base. Legislators and other government officials should be urged to assume more responsibility for this problem since government and the community receive so much of the benefits from gaming" (Bybee 1988, p. 307).

Second, if the gaming industry is going to be forced to make payments for lawsuits against it—as well as forgo debts owed—then the community should be aware of the consequences: smaller casinos, horse tracks, and so on could be forced to shut down, which could jeopardize the economic stability of those cities and states that depend heavily upon a gambling-based income. Bybee (1988) states: "The one common denominator in all of these varied gaming operations is that the public is a substantial direct beneficiary of the gaming proceeds. In many cases, including gaming casinos, the public receives far more in the form of tax revenue than the company earns for its stockholders. Everyone understands the public benefit from state operated lotteries, but many do not understand the extent to which the public gains from privately operated casinos" (p. 302). Bybee (1988) provides an example:

> To illustrate, in 1985, the casinos in Atlantic City produced $2.4 billion in net revenues, retaining only $51.5 million in net profit (2.1%). They paid in direct taxes local, state and federal governments $360.3 million; and they paid an additional $41.2 million regulatory fees. On top of this, $24.1 million, almost half of their profit, was obligated to be reinvested in New Jersey as directed by the Casino Reinvestment Development Authority.
>
> These figures do not include the taxes paid by employees and vendors. Nor do they include the substantial charitable contributions made by some private sector gaming enterprises. (P. 302)

Given the seriousness of these problems, Bybee proposes that the medical field change its conception of the gambler from *pathological* to *problem*. It puts responsibility, rationality, rights, and social and individual justice in their "right" place. This transition in the object of investigation does not mean that gamblers shouldn't receive treatment, or that more research shouldn't be done. What it means is that the right label is applied to the right person: "Problem gamblers should not be punished for having the status of a problem gambler, but they should be held responsible for the consequences of their actions; the responsibility should not be shifted to those who merely provide the opportunity to gamble" (Bybee 1988, p. 304).

The Concerns of the Medical Expert

Obviously Bybee's argument, as well as those of the rest of the gambling industry, were of great concern to the fields of gambling research and treatment during the 1980s and 1990s. Bybee and the gambling industry presented a major counter argument to the medical model—which was slowly beginning to make an important impact. What treatment experts were most concerned about, however, was not the abdication of responsibility. Even though most treatment professionals support the medical model, as the Brecksville pamphlet conveyed, few actually believe that their patients were not responsible for their past actions. What they were most concerned about was the impact Bybee's arguments, and others, would have on the perception of United States society in general. Historically, people were already in general disagreement that gambling was a disease. But now, with the support of the gambling industry, the arguments against the medical model could go too far in the other direction and give the impression that pathological gambling didn't exist at all. What would be the outcome of these arguments? What would become the general perceptions of Americans as the medical model and the gambling industry negotiated their differences?

What Do You Get When You Cross the Medical with the Economic?

The negotiated interactions between the gambling industry and the medical model have resulted in a rather interesting set of discursive arrangements. These arrangements emerged quite by accident through the process of the medical and the economic working together—despite their diverging intentions. The medical and the economic, through their collision, created a set of negotiations which reduced the sociological, political, and economic complexities of pathological gambling to "a problem of individuals."

It started with the treatment professionals. They read the literature, listened to the reports, talked with other experts, and did therapy with recovering gamblers. Across the country, through all of the various knowledge exchanges medical experts had with the rest of the social sciences and the institutions of social control, professionals outside the field started to believe that gambling was perhaps a medical problem. Through these interactions the discourses then moved outward to the general public. This happened as people listened to treatment and research experts on the evening news or in the newspaper. Through these interactions between gambling experts and the general public, gambling started to become recognized as a health care problem. But, because the gambling treatment and research fields never really mounted a campaign against the legalization of gambling the way medicine has attacked the tobacco companies, people in the United States came to believe that gambling was a problem of individuals, just like drug addiction and alcoholism, and not a problem of the community. In other words, the medical model did little to move the general public beyond its previous moral and legal opinion of pathological gambling as a vice that is given in to by largely deviant individuals.

The gambling industry capitalized on this error. At the same time that the medical model was convincing people that gambling was a problem of individuals, the general public was also learning—again through the media and advertising campaigns—that gambling, because it was now legal, was okay to do; something which only a small minority of the population actually had problems with. The larger social consequences were, again, unaddressed. The American public listened to all the commercials and advertisements that gambling was fun and that they could even win, and a growing majority of the population started spending evenings out with friends enjoying a night of gambling or buying their weekly lottery ticket.

Once in a while, however, someone did come out and speak to the social dimensions of the problem. Goodman was one of those people. But, when he published his book, *The Luck Business* (1995), it was largely attacked by the gambling industry as an affront to the freedom of the economic marketplace. Some federal level politicians, such as Frank Wolf, however, did respond by putting together a panel of experts to address the issue. But, nothing really changed. The gambling industry continued to make money and the field of gambling research and treatment continued to use an individualistic, medically reductionistic approach to the problem. Meanwhile, the social consequences of the problem continued to escalate.

Toward the end of the 1990s, however, the negotiations between treatment and research experts and the gambling industry began to get somewhere: representatives from the gambling industry were invited to attend various gambling conferences, and the councils started working with the state lottery commissions to educate the public about the potential dangers of gambling. But why? Why would the gambling industry make such compensations? Why were they suddenly listening to the arguments of the medical experts? Probably because it made good business sense. In the past couple of years, more and more people have been entering treatment, which has started to make the gambling industry look bad. To keep a good image, they've been forced to address the impact legalization has had on society. But, again, only at the level of the individual. The gambling industry still fails to address the economic and social impact gambling has had on our country. And so, as we approach the turn of the century, the gambling industry remains largely unscathed by the frontal attack of the medical model. As a result, these interactions have created a position of negotiated confusion in which people do and do not suffer from the disease of compulsive gambling; people are and are not responsible for their addiction; people should and should not be punished for their problems, and seldom does anyone look at the larger picture to understand the social dimensions of the problem. Until more sociologically minded research is done to clarify this problem, the confusion created by the negotiations between the medical and the economic will more than likely remain.

Chapter 9

GOVERNMENT

Obtainment of political, institutional, organizational, legal, and cultural position up to this point, both in the forms of medical treatment and economics, has been through obsessive attention to the details of discourse.[1] Through their negotiations, business and treatment have waged campaigns (mostly in opposition to one another) in an effort to make certain things known to people. Making things heard, making noise, drawing attention to new ways of thinking about gambling—these have been the obsessive concerns of business and treatment in the games of "truth" surrounding pathological gambling. As the games have played themselves out during the 1980s and 1990s, the various discursive actors involved have gone to great lengths to carve out the necessary concepts, theories, empirical findings, legal evidence, and key objects of investigation upon which to ground their perspectives; all in an effort to convince others to think differently so that the medical model and the gambling industry can continue on with their objectives.

The techniques used to accomplish these objectives have rarely been spelled out with full conscious intent. Rather, they have emerged in a reactionary manner as a function of the discursive strategies themselves. The discourses of business and treatment are chameleon like; they change as is necessary to accommodate the field of negotiations they happen to be struggling within. This is not to suggest that deceit is their primary objective; many of the actors involved believe in what they are doing. The necessary act of subjectified discursive negotiation requires them to resolve their own discursive incongruence, be it in favor of or against legalization. We all preach what we believe. And we convert others so they may believe as well.

It is the obsessiveness with discourse on the part of business and treatment that makes the acts of government so strange. Government, both at the state and federal level, has waged its campaign on pathological gambling by primarily remaining silent, by refusing to articulate a discourse, stance, or major position. To government's credit, there are a few state level initiatives that are beginning to support the study and treatment of pathological gambling, along with support for helplines, public awareness, and epidemiological studies, as in Maryland, where legislators have worked with Dr. Lorenz and colleagues for the past several years. But, these are few and far between. Most states have done nothing. It is this odd approach to pathological gambling that makes the role of government in these negotiations uniquely important.

Consider the role of government in the United States. Its objective is to govern, to care for, and to represent the needs and desires of its people. Congress and the various states pass laws, enact policies, sign contracts, draw up agreements, activate programs, construct organizations, and so on. In each of these activities a discourse is necessary. Without writing up the goals and objectives of a law or program, nobody knows how to vote or put them into practice. Government must make its objectives known by constructing a discourse which explains to others how and why people should act a certain way. Without the discourse, no action takes place.

Awareness of the fact that *no discourse means no action* has been the basis for the major social activists of this century. It wasn't until people were instructed in certain alternative discourses that they came to recognize at a national level that, for example, spousal abuse and racism are wrong. Without discourses on poverty, equal rights, capitalism, religion, and democracy—republican, democrat, or third-party—it would be impossible to obtain the level of negotiated agreement necessary to govern. Action would be impossible. If a discourse doesn't exist, then neither does the phenomena that it was meant to bring to life.

In the case of pathological gambling, the failure on the part of state and federal governments to construct an explicit discourse on the problems of pathological gambling has resulted in nation-wide ignorance about pathological gambling and its problems. People know that gambling is now legal but they don't really know why or how. Most people are also aware—

as I explained in the previous chapter—that excessive gambling can result in problems and that there's medical treatment for it. But why this treatment is medical in nature is beyond them—even professionals within mental health and the social sciences lack this knowledge. How is it, then, that pathological gambling, as defined by treatment, has become a major social problem in the United States, affecting millions of people, and yet the majority of our politicians give the impression that they are completely unaware of this problem? The answer: money and a lack of discursive strategies within which to issue complaint.

On the whole, our United States Government, both at the state and federal level, has specifically neglected to construct a discourse (and, therefore, implement the appropriate programs, policies, or laws) about pathological gambling because it is incongruent with the general intentions and beliefs of their "for-profit," pro-gambling discourses. Certainly, some would disagree because there are politicians working to deal with the problems of pathological gambling, and some states are specifically anti-gambling. That is true. To a certain extent, government's role in gambling depends upon the city or state in question. In states like Louisiana or New Jersey, for example, the government is ardently pro-gambling, but in states like Utah, the government has been strictly anti-gambling. You also have to contend with differences between the federal and state level. Some politicians have spoken out about the need to address gambling as a social problem. Regardless, because every state short of Utah and Hawaii have some form of legalized gambling, and because over twenty three states have some form of casino gambling, be it river boat gambling or land casinos, it is safe to say that the dominant trend in government has been definitely pro-gambling. If politicians are to survive in our current economic climate, they must find ways to generate revenue. Gambling provides this promise. In 1997, for example, Iowa made nearly $160 million from gambling,[2] and at a national level, combined state profits were over $10 billion.[3]

The problem with the "for-profit," pro-gambling discourses isn't that government shouldn't allow people to gamble. The problem is that, in doing so, government has put itself in a dangerous position which jeopardizes the very role of government itself. Goodman (1995) explains: "In the case of gambling, it is the government which is explicitly trying to get people to participate more, through advertisements, media promotions, and public relations campaigns. It is the government which is expanding the availability of more addictive forms of gambling like electronic gambling machines. The result is a dangerous shift in the fundamental role of government—from regulator of gambling to promoter of gambling" (p. 135).

For the first time in United States history, government is not trying to regulate business or work to help business make a profit. Government is actually in the business of business itself. When it comes to gambling, government is a business. But a business more powerful than any other. In our country, the government is supposed to hold business in check through regulation, not act in the capacity of business. The problem is that when government is both business and regulator, it is easy to manipulate regulations to accommodate the drive for profit. The boundaries between business and government become blurred. In states where gambling is legalized, government is in contradiction with itself. In their new role, pro-gambling politicians, and their committees and organizations, negotiate with the general public to increase their level of gambling. State sponsored gambling commercials inundate the television and print media, telling people: Play the lottery and win a new car. Vote to legalize gambling to support your school systems. Help to elect a mayor who is pro-gambling, because pro-gambling is pro-jobs. We promise to bring in 1,000 new jobs by implementing six new river boats. On and on the campaign goes. Government, disguising itself as government, tricks people into believing they are listening to government when, in fact, people are really listening to just another manifestation of the gambling industry. Goodman (1995) states:

> While people have always dreamed of a lucky break in a card game or perhaps picking a winning number, never before have they been so blatantly urged by their political leaders to risk their money in order to transform the declining situation of their lives. What began as a reasonable effort to capture, for the public coffers, dollars already being bet illegally has mushroomed into an enterprise that is radically transforming the role of government. . . . [That we have] arrived at a point in time where state government agencies are studying demographics and psychological behavior of state residents in order to encourage them to gamble more, not only raises serious moral questions, but calls for a more fundamental reassessment of the nature of government's role in the business of gambling. (P. 155)

Because of the enormous profits being made by the government, most politicians and their committees give the impression that they have ignored the problems of pathological gambling. Of the number of ways to illustrate this, I will consider one: the war on drugs versus the war on gambling.

My argument is as follows: while the government wages a war on drugs, it's at peace with pathological gambling because gambling sustains the government economically. If the government started a war on pathological gambling, it would have to consider itself one of its primary enemies and make accomodations to both allow people to gamble while providing services to those who fall prey to its problems.

Everybody knows about the war on drugs in the United States. And everyone is vaguely familiar with the controversy and the arguments back and forth about drug legalization and the Drug War's failures. Since the 1980s, the United States government has spent billions and billions of dollars fighting drugs. The annual expenditure of public money is about $70 billion.[4] Our borders are policed, pushers are arrested and users are imprisoned—conservative estimates suggest that 50 percent of the prisoners in jail are there because of drug related crimes.[5] Governmentally funded treatment centers, which the Substance Abuse and Mental Health Services Administration (SAMHSA, www.samhsa.gov) helps to organize and interact with, exist everywhere throughout the country and are almost too numerous to even count. Government campaigns such as DARE (Drug Abuse Resistance Education) and organizations like the American Council for Drug Education (www.acde.org) have gone into communities, the schools, and the workplace to educate adults and children that drugs are bad. Since the Reagan years, when the war first started, each president has made drugs a primary focus. Bush appointed drug czar William Bennett to run the Office of National Drug Control Policy and Clinton appointed retired General Barry McCaffrey to implement his National Drug Control Strategy.[6] Research institutions, which receive billions of dollars annually from government to provide new information on drug usage and treatment, were also established. The most important institutions include the National Institute on Drug Abuse (NIDA, www.nida. nih.gov) and the National Institute on Alcoholism and Alcohol Abuse (NIAAA, www.niaaa. nih.gov). NIDA and NIAAA are both part of the National Institutes of Health (NIH). State-level organizations include the National Association of State Alcohol and Drug Abuse Directors (www.nasadad.org), UCLA Drug Abuse Research Center (www.mednet.ucla.edu/ som/ddo/npi/DARC), and the Indiana Prevention Resource Center (www.drugs.indiana.edu).

As a result of government's war on drugs and its involvement in creating funding and supporting state organizations, institutions, and programs throughout the country, people across the United States have become "educated" about the drug problem. Government, at the state and federal level, has gone to incredible lengths to create the needed concepts, theories, and empirical findings to convince us that drugs are bad. In short, because government wanted to do something about drugs, discourses were created so that action could take place. Policy was initiated, and change (for good and bad) occurred. Contrast this heavy involvement in drugs with the peace treatise on gambling.

Even though the "drug problem" and pathological gambling both became politically important social issues at the beginning of the 1980s, there currently exists only one federally funded grant in the United States for the study of the problems of pathological gambling. It is part of the Healthy People 2000 Initiative and is in conjunction with NIH, NIDA, and NIAAA. The title of the grant is "Pathological Gambling: Basic, Clinical and Service Research." The grant is offered in conjunction with the only (private) national center to offer funding for the study of pathological gambling, The National Center for Responsible Gaming (NCRG), which is a non-profit organization put together by the Gaming Entertainment Research and Education Foundation, whose board members include representatives of the gaming industry and leaders from the field of gambling research and treatment, the public, the service sector, and other charitable organizations.

Other than this one grant (which is a major step forward) and the few state initiatives which provide money for counseling and gambling hotline services, there is almost no other money specifically set aside—only about $18 million[7]—by the government to address the problems of pathological gambling: there are no federally funded programs going into the communities or school systems educating people about the dangers of excessive gambling; no gambling czars; no federally appointed commissioners; no agency patrolling the borders or running to protect the children and family members of pathological gamblers; there is nothing. All that exists are a handful of state-level councils, of which only a few are highly organized and ready.

Even the currently existing governmental programs for drug abuse research and treatment, such as NIDA, do not provide in-depth funding for pathological gambling—as mentioned, only one grant currently exists. They even ignore the issue of gambling comorbidity. In a recent study of 944 patients admitted to in-patient treatment for pathological gambling, 33 percent reported past or current addiction to alcohols or drugs, and 52 percent had a comorbid psychiatric disorder.[8]

Because pathological gambling is largely ignored and few state councils have any money, researchers are left to their own devices to find the financial support needed to do in-depth research. So, they turn to one of the two places where money is available: the gambling industry (as in the case of NCRG) or the pharmaceutical companies. Turning to the gambling industry, researchers are put in a position where they may have to compromise their discourses against gambling in order to "do business." When they interact with the pharmaceutical companies, their work becomes even more medicalized. The gambling treatment facilities are in the same position. They must rely upon private support to fuel their programs. Because they have to find ways to stay in business, they then turn to the medical discourse because it is the most powerful discourse available to argue the need for money from insurance companies and HMO's.

While the federal government has remained silent on the issue of pathological gambling, a discourse may finally be on its way. Thanks to the efforts of Congressman Frank Wolf, the National Gambling Impact Study Commission (www.ngisc.gov) was enacted in 1996. Since its inception, however, it has been engulfed in controversy. In fact, the commission didn't get under way until 1997 because of the politics surrounding the appointment of the commission's panel members.

The current board consists of Kay James (Chair and Dean of the Robertson School of Government), William Bible (Chairman of the Nevada State Gaming Control), James Dobson (a psychologist who is famous for his Christian radio program, Focus on the Family), Terrence Lanni (Chairman of the Board and CEO of MGM Grand Inc.), Richard Leone (President of the Twentieth Century Fund), Robert Loescher (President and CEO of Sealaska Corporation), Leo McCarthy (Former Lieutenant Governor of California), Paul Harold Moore (physician and founding member and President of Singing River Radiology Group), and John Wilhelm (General Secretary and Treasurer for the Hotel Employees & Restaurant Employees International Union). Notably missing from the panel is a single expert in the field of gambling research or treatment.

The sub-panel put together by the Committee for the Study of Pathological Gambling includes the following: Rachel Volberg (President of Gemini Research), Howard Shaffer (Director of the Center for Addiction

Studies at Harvard Medical School and Editor of the Journal of Gambling Studies), Henry Lesieur (Institute for Problem Gambling), Valerie Lorenz (Executive Director of the Compulsive Gambling Center), Edward Looney (Executive Director of the Counsel on Compulsive Gambling), and Arnold Wexler (President of Arnie & Sheila Wexler Associates). This sub-panel met with members of the main panel on 22 January 1998.

The National Gambling Impact Study Commission Act was formed in response to the federal government's absolute lack of both knowledge and action regarding the social, economic, and psychological consequences of legalized gambling. The last federal study completed was in 1976. At the time, few states had legalized gambling, and the study only focused on gambling in two states over a three year period. Recognizing that so much had changed since then, a new commission was put into action.

The goals of the committee are as follows. First, they are to review existing state and federal laws and policies and practices with respect to the legalization and prohibition of gambling. Second, they are to assess issues related to gambling and crime. Third, they are to review issues related to problem and pathological gambling. Fourth, they are to assess the impact legalized gambling has had on the psychological, familial, cultural, and economic situations of communities throughout the United States, particularly as these consequences relate to advertising and promotion of gambling. Fifth, they are to explore the revenue made by states as a result of gambling and what other alternatives may be used to generate this income, and, sixth, examine the latest forms of electronic gambling (including the Internet) and the interstate and international impact of gambling legalization. The outcome of the study will be released toward the end of 1999. Until then, our federal and state level government is without discursive voice in a cacophony of opinions and arguments.

Because government has largely remained silent on the issue, pathological gambling *literally* remains a *hidden epidemic*. Through its powers of persuasion, government's lack of involvement has limited people's knowledge across the country during the 1980s and 1990s to a "watered down" awareness that gambling is probably a medical problem that certain deviant individuals suffer from, but is okay for most people to participate in since it's legal. Besides, the government hasn't declared it a major social problem yet. It will, therefore, be interesting to see what happens once the NGISC report comes out.

Chapter 10

DIAGNOSED PATHOLOGICAL GAMBLERS

It is important to recognize that, at the time of Torniero's trial, while experts on behalf of both the defense and the prosecution were brought in to battle it out, the voices of those whose lives were actually affected by the problems and excesses of gambling were not present. The voices not present totaled three: pathological gamblers, inveterate gamblers, and the families and friends of these people.

Viewed together, what is interesting about these three voices is that during the 1980s and 1990s, they held few common assumptions about pathological gambling. What united them, instead, was their common struggle to resolve the opposing arguments raised by the defense and the prosecution. They were in a difficult situation. They had to negotiate a discursive response to the questions of responsibility and rights, rehabilitation and punishment. And, it had to be adequate enough to defend or heal their position in life. Pathological gamblers went one way, inveterate gamblers went another. Families and friends were somewhere in the middle, hoping that their own struggles and suffering would receive attention as well.

Given the common struggle of these three positions, two questions immediately emerge. First of all, how and why did these three different forces come to their different conclusions about the medical model of pathological gambling? Was it a function of their understanding of the clinical and legal literature or were there personal, cultural, political, and economic factors involved as well? Second, what were the consequences of their different conclusions? How did their decisions impact their lives and the lives of those around them? To answer these questions, we start with the pathological gambler.

The Making of the Pathological Gambler

After thirty days of treatment, patients leave the Brecksville Gambling Treatment Program. On the day of discharge they take the elevator to the first floor and exit the building. Standing on the sidewalk, they look to their left, then to their right. They can go in any direction. It's their choice. They've come to the end of one life ready to begin another. In their suitcase reside the tools for recovery: GA pamphlets, phone numbers for aftercare counselors and a sponsor, conceptions of the disease model and the twelve-step program, theories about their neuropsychological makeup, and general treatment advice given since Custer. They have negotiated long and hard for thirty days. They've been challenged, broken down, questioned, built up, and supported. Now they are ready to do it on their own. Medical discourse in hand, they are ready to re-negotiate their lives, ready to change themselves from a gambling failure to a medical winner.

So how do these diagnosed pathological gamblers re-negotiate their lives? How do they handle the difficult issues of responsibility and right, punishment and rehabilitation? To answer these questions, I will explore the confessions of three diagnosed pathological gamblers. All three confessions were published in Rose's (1988) special edition of the *Journal of Gambling Studies*. What makes these confessions important is that all three authors were not only diagnosed pathological gamblers, but had also been charged with some form of gambling related crime and were either doing time in jail or had just gotten out. The arguments made by the medical model and those in opposition to it—as in the case of Torniero's trial—were, therefore, central to their writings.

Let the Negotiations Begin

Ottinger

> It was summer. I was five years old. The corn which grew up to the back yard, where I was playing with my three-year-

old brother, was not "as high as an elephant's eye" (the red clay of eastern Tennessee was not as productive as the alluvial loam of Oklahoma); but it was tall enough to conceal my father as he crept up to the back of the house.

I ran to tell my mother that father was home. Mother and her cousin were adjusting their clothing.

Father divorced mother. In those good old days (1920) adultery was considered such a stain on a woman's character (but not on a man's), that the custody of me and my brother was given to Father without argument. He did not want us, but he did want revenge. He was later charged with child neglect but acquitted when he gave us back to our mother, temporarily.

We thought she did not want us, either.

How does one become a compulsive gambler? With this kind of background, it doesn't seem to be hard.

When I was 15 years old, I lost all my paper route money in my first poker game. I was so annoyed with my lack of self-control, that I promised myself that I would never gamble again; and I didn't, until I attended baby judge's school in Reno 43 years later, when I lost all my extra money in the slot machines.

Again, I made the same promise. I kept it for fifteen years. By then I was so heavily in debt (a divorce and remarriage, two families to support, three children to put through college, a contested double campaign, an inadequate judicial salary), with my judgement impaired by alcohol, that I tried to recoup by gambling. There were three state lotteries and two race tracks within easy reach; and there were numerous accommodating poker playing friends. Winning was exhilarating; losing was hell. After a while I was gambling to get the rush, like a runner's high, which accompanies the gambling itself, regardless of winning or losing.

Of course I knew that using the money of others was wrong, but I could not seem to stop. There came a Friday when I knew I would have to produce $50,000 on Monday. I did not have it and I could not get it.

I disappeared for three months.

I was arrested in April 1987 and have been in jail ever since. In federal court my crimes were called mail fraud. In the state court the same incidents were labeled forgery and larceny. . . .

After a great deal of sober reflection (I stopped drinking entirely seven weeks before I was incarcerated), I have concluded that compulsive gambling is an illness (or a disease, as lawyers prefer), just as alcoholism and drug dependency are illnesses. (Ottinger 1988, pp. 309–310)

Paul

My name is Paul. I am an investment banker, financial advisor, attorney, certified public accountant, former federal agent, husband, father, grandfather, and, oh yes, a recovering compulsive gambler. I made my last bet on April 14, 1982, the same day that a jury of my peers found me guilty of five felony counts for passing bad checks in Las Vegas, Nevada. Until that time I truly believed I could control my gambling habit and thought I was too smart to be a compulsive gambler. Apparently the jury reached the same conclusion in their guilty verdict. When polled after the trial, the jury foreman stated "they were of the opinion that Mr. A. was too intelligent a person to really be a compulsive gambler."

At the suggestion of my defense counsel, I attended several Gamblers Anonymous meetings prior to the date of my conviction, and I sought the advice and medical assistance of experts in the field of compulsive gambling, only to find their conclusion was that, in fact, I was a "compulsive gambler." Not until after my conviction was I able to take the First Step of the GA Recovery Program—I realized and admitted to myself that I was powerless over gambling—and that my life had become unmanageable. At the same time I had to face the rude awakening that I was suspended from the practice of law, my license to practice as a certified public accountant would also be suspended, and a major real estate company I had worked so hard to develop would ultimately be dismantled by the bankruptcy courts.

After a year and a half of appeals my unblemished record of the past would be marred by a conviction which the United States Supreme Court denied review, and which led to my incarceration on November 28, 1983. Although I had never had a prior conviction, I was facing a sentence of three years in prison which, in the words of the federal judge who rendered that sentence, "was the only way I would stop gambling. . . ."

After filing 172 different motions, affidavits, petitions, briefs, and after many hours of prayer and meditation, relief was finally granted in February 1984, when the trial court agreed to review my case. At the time and once again with the help of GA and my sponsor, the judge reviewing my case concurred that I was a compulsive gambler, and that a reduction in my sentence would be appropriate. Finally, after several months of review, I was released from prison on August 22, 1984. (A. Paul 1988, pp. 312–313)

Jarvis

When I was about ten, on July 26, 1952, my father took my mother and me fishing. My dad rented a boat while my mother and I stayed on the beach. Then we went out in a boat, too, to be with Dad. When we got close to the bridge where he was, we saw him pulling up the anchor. His boat was rocking from the waves made by a passing power boat, and my father fell in. He splashed for a minute, and then he went under and never came up again. My mother stood screaming. I couldn't swim and neither could my dad.

There must have been 20 people on shore fishing about 20 yards away, but no one went to help him. My mother kept screaming and holding on to me.

Later, when they found my father's body, they put him in a bag and put him on the floor of a garage next to a fire station. I could see him through a window. It looked so cold in there. I ran away and the police found me that night walking down a highway. They brought me back to my mother, but I kept running away. I would run away and the police would catch me and bring me to Juvenile Home. I was there 31 times. At least that is the last count I can remember. Wherever they sent me, I would run away. This kept up until they sent me to state reformatory. I tried to commit suicide there by cutting my wrist. They gave me 81 stitches.

> I started gambling about this time. When I got out, I worked, but lost my money gambling in Vegas. After that it was just work, gamble, write bad checks, go to prison, get out and start all over again. This is the sixth time.
>
> I am taking some counseling courses now in prison, hoping to learn about myself and also to help me get a job when I get out. You suggested I see a prison psychologist, but I don't think that they have a psychologist here. At least I haven't heard of any. . . .
>
> You asked me if I thought compulsive gambling is an illness. Yes, it definitely is. I believe it is both a physical and mental illness. In the same way an addict feels the physical need for dope, I have felt the need to get more money to gamble after I had lost what money I had. . . . I know I need treatment, but I don't know exactly what kind. (Jarvis 1988, p. 317–318)

Medical Confession and the Act of Telling the Truth

We are presented with three texts. Ottinger and Jarvis write their letters from the prison cell. Paul from the outside. All three men are trying to save their lives. Ottinger, a former judge, is 73 years old. Instead of enjoying the final years of his life, he is dying in jail. Paul is trying to rebuild his career as a lawyer, real-estate agent, and financial planner. He is having very little success. Jarvis has no life. But, he is hoping to find one. In an effort to find some relief, perhaps even some sympathy, all three men took the time to write out their lives to explain why they did what they did. They are desperate men writing to make a difference, a difference in the way we think about them. Perhaps they can change our understanding of them. At least they are going to try.

To change our discursive understanding of them, all three men engage in the act of medicalized confession. But why medicalized confession? Why not some other technique or perspective?

Medical Confession as a Technique of Inquiry

In contemporary society, the social sciences are a primary provider of the "truths" necessary to help our institutions of social control (e.g., the criminal justice system, the prison, the mental health facility, etc) maintain varying degrees of social order—particularly over social problems like pathological gambling.

To uncover the "truth" about various social problems, social scientists have developed a number of important techniques and practices. Examples of these practices include survey research, psychometric testing, biopsychosocial assessment, ethnography, participant observation, structured and unstructured interviewing, therapy, and written biography. In the field of gambling treatment, one of the most useful practices is the act of medical confession. Addiction counselors generally believe that the only way to salvation, to health, to freedom from gambling, is through a thorough examination of the innermost places of the patient's mind and soul. All secrets must be exposed and revealed for what they are. Only by exposing the secrets and the inner workings of the patient can the "truth" about her or his addiction be determined. Once these "hidden truths" are revealed, the pathological gambler must speak them openly. It is through the act of public confession that normalcy is restored and the gambling failure can return to the status of winner. Gamblers Anonymous does this as well. Every night, throughout the country, people stand up and confess the "truth" about themselves in hopes that the act of confession will keep them on the path of recovery. They are scared for their lives; they hope they get it right. If they relapse, they rework their story to tell it better. They have to get the story right, and so back to the beginning they go, telling the story once again.

Within the context of a theory of discursive negotiations, the act of confession is a complicated act. While Foucault (1979) argues that practices such as confession are ways in which the institutions of social control—via the social sciences—gain a position of dominance over the guilty, he fails to understand the ways in which those who must confess likewise manipulate the system for their own individual agendas. In short, he fails to understand both the two-fold nature of interaction and the "negotiated" nature of confession. The negotiated act of confession requires us to understand that confession is more than just a technique used by various institutions, such as prisons or hospitals, to dominate and control patients. It is also a technique by which patients and prisoners gain control over their own lives and the institutions in which they live. Therefore, if they are going to be useful, most confessional techniques, such as written biography, testing, and interviewing, require a number of important negotiated agreements between staff and patients. Confession is, therefore, always already an act of negotiation which is engaged in by specific subjectified agents (pathological gamblers) involved in the two-fold process of interaction comprising the organizing practices (primarily the medical model) in which they live.

Medical Confession and Its Negotiated Benefits

The benefits of the negotiated act of medical confession are as follows:

1. Staff and institution use the negotiated act of confession to gain control over patients by exposing their internal workings. If staff know the innermost secrets of patients, then they can manipulate their vulnerabilities to push them in certain directions. They obtain a position of control and dominance that can be used to heal or hurt. And so, they are always prodding patients to reveal more.

2. Staff and the institution also use confession as a way to protect and help patients in the world outside of treatment. They use the insights of their profession to lobby for political, economic, and cultural change in our conceptions of addiction, illness, and pathology. If they tell patients that confessing will help others like them, patients are more likely to talk.

3. Staff and the institution also use confession to either uphold or deny mainstream values of what it means to be healthy and what it means to be addicted. Treatment experts can reinforce our current war on drugs and our conceptions of gambling addiction, or challenge these perspectives to construct new ways of understanding and treating addiction. Depending upon the objective of the treatment expert, they can use confession to push clients in different moral directions. Under the pressure of a powerful therapist, for example, clients may give in and accept a morality different from their own. It all depends on how the game is played out.

4. In terms of patients, they use confession to clarify their situation in hopes that explaining themselves will free them from the control and domination of the institution. For example, if a patient confesses, he can show the staff that he is working to make a difference in his life. The staff, in turn, label the patient as a "good patient" and reward him for his good behavior. The patient, however, is only confessing to manipulate and control the opinions of staff so he can get a good letter of recommenda-

tion, or perhaps so he can get his wife or his job back—and then get back to gambling.

5. Patients also hope that confession will resolve them of a certain amount of responsibility for their past, which likewise frees them from control and domination. If the patient confesses that she has a disease, then she is freed of a certain amount of responsibility. In the eyes of society, she suffers from a sickness, not a failure in moral character.

6. Patients use confession to obtain various objectives in their relationships with others outside treatment, such as spouses, family, friends, employers, the criminal justice system and society in general. Wedgeworth (1998) explains that the leading factor influencing a pathological gambler's admission to the hospital is a strained relationship with a significant other, employer, or criminal justice system. It is hardly ever the gambling by itself. We must realize, then, that most patients are not in treatment just to stop the gambling. They are in treatment to fix a relationship. If stopping their gambling is part of fixing the relationship, then that is what they will do—at least for a while.

7. Patients use confession as a way to change themselves into something other than what they currently are in hopes that they can gain back a sense of control over their lives; with this control comes happiness, peace, and various other desires and objectives. A certain percentage of patients, about one out of three, are in treatment to change. These patients use confession as a technique of self exploration. They believe that complete honesty is necessary if they are to change their lives.

8. Lastly, patients use confession to lobby for cultural, political, institutional, and economic change. Through their confessions they challenge the addiction treatment staff and society to view their problems differently or obtain various freedoms and levels of authority and position. While few patients do become activists, there are those who do. In the public arena, their authority comes from their life experiences. They use confession as the technique to obtain this power.

Ottinger, Paul, and Jarvis and the Act of Medical Confession

Given our general understanding of the act of medical confession, it is now time to examine how Ottinger, Paul, and Jarvis used this technique to argue a case on their behalf. Our examination of their usage of medical confession will be broken down into two primary sections: 1) the discursive negotiations they have with others and 2) the negotiations they have with themselves. It is important to understand that medical confession works both toward the self and toward others. In other words, because of the interpretive and inter-active nature of confession, how and why pathological gamblers confess to others the "truth" about themselves may not necessarily have a direct relation to what they believe and confess to themselves. The game of confession is therefore a delicate balance between the ways in which each of us presents ourselves to others, versus the way we view ourselves in the privacy of our own minds. We start with the gambler's negotiations with others.

The medical model has made its way, a long journey, from the Brecksville, VA, and other treatment centers throughout the country into the letters of Ottinger, Paul, and Jarvis. It has negotiated its way into their understandings of themselves. They have used it to help them make certain things known in order to get certain things done. In this case, they have used the medical model to resolve the following question: if someone commits a crime because she has an illness, should you punish or rehabilitate her? These three men think, based on the medical model, that punishment is a waste of time and rehabilitation the only solution.

To accomplish their negotiation, these men make the same two-pronged argument Keefe made in Torniero's pre-trial hearing. First, relying upon their own personal struggles and the insights of treatment experts, they argue that they suffer from an illness, an illness severe enough for them to commit a crime. Paul states, "Yes, I was a lawyer who had committed wrongs. Had I ever done anything similar before? No. Do I believe that compulsive gambling is an illness? Yes, I know what it did to my ability to reason. I would not have ever considered such criminal behavior had I not lost control over my gambling" (A. Paul 1988, pp. 314–315).

Like the experts brought in on behalf of the defense, these men testify to the irrational, impulsive, erratic, and "insane" behavior caused when pathological gamblers start "chasing" their losses and cannot "win back" control over their lives. They go out of their minds. They are no longer the same person, as if they're under a spell which they cannot break until they've destroyed everything. Jarvis states, "You asked me if I thought compulsive gambling is an illness. Yes, it definitely is. I believe it is both a physical and a mental illness. In the same way an addict feels the physical need for dope, I have felt the need to get more money to gamble after I had lost what money I had. . . . I would stop gambling only when I went broke or out of sheer exhaustion" (1988, p. 318).

Because they suffer from an illness, according to Paul, Ottinger and Jarvis, punishing them and sending them to prison does nothing but make it worse. Now they've been stigmatized with a criminal record and, losing dignity and self respect, it becomes even harder for them to recover some type of life. The failure of punishment to help pathological gamblers leads to the second prong of the argument made by these three men: punishment does not change the behaviors of a pathological gambler, only rehabilitation does.

Paul states, "Do I believe that I should have been punished by incarceration? No. I believe a better resolution would have been the requirement to perform community service, to take public responsibility for my conduct, to enter treatment for rehabilitation to prevent further gambling or further conduct, and to make restitution to those who had been defrauded by me" (A. Paul 1988, p. 315). Like Jarvis and Ottinger, Paul feels that he could have paid his debt to society in a more useful way, in a way that would have helped both him and his victims. He states, "I believe my incarceration resulted not only in unnecessary expense to the state, but great deprivation to my family, who were, after all, also victims of my mental disorder. Through required community service I would have been able to continue to support my family, pay back gambling debts, and certainly would have benefited from the services I could have provided to them" (A. Paul 1988, p. 315).

Ottinger makes a similar argument. He states, "Is incarceration useful under these circumstances?" His response: "For a short time perhaps. Something drastic needs to be done, no doubt, to break the addictive habit pattern, but jail for more than a few months is a waste of public funds and the talent of the defendant" (1988, p. 310). While the arguments these men present make sense, they do pose a serious challenge to the criminal justice system in the United States. If rehabilitation is the goal of the courtroom in these instances, what happens to justice? What happens to punishment? What prevents crime from becoming a disease? With these types of arguments, these men travel the same precipice as Custer and Milt (1985) did when they *pathologized* the criminal behavior of pathological gamblers. If all criminal behavior is a manifestation of some psychological or social pathology, then why punish anyone?

Jarvis has a potential solution: punishment for a short time, but rehabilitation in the long run. Jarvis states, "Do I think that the compulsive gambler who commits crimes should be punished by incarceration? I believe that if a person commits a crime for whatever reason that he should pay for it. But I also believe that the punishment should not be emphasized so much as the treatment. Punishment will not stop a person from gambling whereas treatment will. Then the person won't do the same thing over and over again" (Jarvis 1988, p. 319).

If Jarvis was admitted to the psychiatric ward instead of a prison, he would probably be diagnosed with Post Traumatic Stress Disorder. Watching his father die was too much. Jarvis broke down and never fully recovered. He let go of life to spend his days floating unhappily behind the sky. He was imprisoned six times, each and every one of them for writing bad checks. He would get caught and thrown in jail. He would get out, work for a while, but then start gambling again. He would write bad checks, get caught again, and go to jail. Finally, the sixth time in jail someone gave him some attention. He finally got the help he deserved from the beginning. Jarvis is grateful, but not negligent. He states:

> A person is supposedly incarcerated for the purposes of protecting the public. Incarceration alone does not do this unless treatment is given. Most offenders do not recognize that they have a problem unless it is pointed out to them. About 25 percent of the people I have met in prison should be in prison indefinitely, the other 75 percent had a problem that could be corrected with some kind of treatment.
>
> I guess the first and hardest thing is to get the person to recognize that he has a problem. All my life I thought that my problem with gambling was losing. My teacher pointed out what my problem was and after being honest with myself I recognized that compulsive gambling is an illness itself, and losing is just a symptom. I am trying to learn more about this so that I can understand it.
>
> We are unable to order books through the library here, and they don't have the books that you recommended. They also do not have a Gamblers Anonymous in this prison. I do want to receive help and make this my last time in jail. Perhaps I can do this—with the help of others who understand compulsive gambling. I know I can't do it alone. (P. 319)

Overall, the letters of Ottinger, Paul, and Jarvis show us that patients are not passive recipients of their discursive environments. The discursive relationship between pathological gamblers, the medical model and the prison system are much more negotiated than that. They do not simply *take on* the ideas, concepts, and treatments doctors prescribe. Even in situations where a doctor is completely totalitarian, the pathological gambler still makes the decision whether or not to follow through with treatment. In mental health for example, "about one third of all patients comply with treatment, one third sometimes comply with certain aspects of treatment, and one third never comply with treatment. An overall figure assessed from a number of studies indicated that 54 percent of patients comply with treatment at any given time" (Kaplan, Sadock and Grebb 1994, p. 11). And so, again, we have another reason why only about one-in-three pathological gamblers are gambling free at one-year post-treatment. It has to do with finding a balance between responsibility and rights, freedom and justice, rehabilitation and punishment.

The perspective within sociology that views the doctor/patient relationship as a give-and-take interaction has been labeled by Uta Gerhardt (1989) as the *negotiation model*. The primary theoretical advocate of this position is Anselm Strauss (1978, 1993). According to Strauss (1978), in an effort to get things done, actors—be they nations, organizations, doctors or patients—must constantly come to some sort of agreement. These agreements, no matter how hostile or conflictual, require actors at some level to bargain with one another, concede, give-in, make concessions, alter plans, change position, accommodate one another and so on. Any act which has as its primary purpose the obtainment of some level of agreement, be it for however long—two minutes, two months, two years—Strauss defines under the heading of negotiation (1978):

> The framework in question has been termed the "negotiated order perspective." It recognizes and attempts to take into account the importance of understanding interaction processes as well as the structural features of organizational life. It stresses the point of view that one of the principal ways that things get accomplished in organizations is through people negotiating with one another, and it takes the theoretical position that both individual action and organizational constraint can be

> comprehended by understanding the nature and contexts of those negotiations. (Maines and Charleton 1985, pp. 271–272)

The important difference negotiation brings to our understanding of the pathological gambler is the sense that the discourses we make known in our daily lives in order to get things done are always being *worked at,* are in process, are never quite finished. They require various levels of complicit and explicit agreement and compromise. In short, discourse is forever in negotiation; we are forever in discursive negotiation. The idea of discursive negotiation is very different from the work of Foucault. In Foucault's work, there is always the sense that the *other,* the patient, the *resisting* actor engaged in the game of domination, is never really "working things out" as much as she is "taking things on." Foucault states:

> Max Weber posed the question: If one wants to behave rationally and regulate one's action according to true principles, what part of one's self should one renounce? What is the ascetic price of reason? To what kind of asceticism should one submit? I posed the opposite question: How have certain kinds of interdictions required the price of certain kinds of knowledge about oneself? What must one know about oneself in order to be willing to renounce anything? (1988, p .17)

Weber's question is closer to the idea of "working things out," while Foucault's question focuses on "taking things on." Foucault dismisses the idea that individuals are comprised of a series of competing discourses or that actors are always already more than the discourses being brought down upon them. Instead, actors are blank discursive slates that engage in an act of domination over themselves. Through the act of domination they come to an understanding of themselves. They are not discovering some deep internal truth. Instead, they are applying a new discourse that changes how they view the "truth" about themselves and the worlds in which they live. A pathological gambler who goes into treatment and finds out he has a disease isn't discovering the "truth" about himself. He has adopted the medical discourse which explains this to him. Once applied, "taken on," the gambler is ready to renounce most other 'truths" or competing discourses about himself.

While I agree with Foucault that "truth" is not so much discovered as it is applied, the act of application is more interactive (as we saw in our review of discursive agency in chapter five). Pathological gamblers do not walk into an in-patient medical treatment center one day and come out two months later "willing to renounce anything else" because of the disciplinary processes of medicalization. The gamblers I worked with came into treatment ready to negotiate, ready to compromise, ready to make accommodations, bargain. They often had a specific agenda, and were there to use treatment to make certain things known about themselves. Because they were often scared and in trouble with family, friends, bookies, bosses, and the law, a good percentage of them were very manipulative and dominating. They manipulated staff, the police, lawyers, and other patients to get what they needed. I saw staff and employers respond to the manipulations of gamblers by making exceptions, altering policy, and re-negotiating their approaches to treatment. And yet, in the midst of the manipulation, most patients struggled to change their lives. They knew something was wrong and wanted help fixing it. They felt that their lives were out of control and wanted to do something about it. It was because of their complicated presentation in treatment that I found it difficult to see them only as merely recipients of the medical model. Perhaps other populations would better fit the passive victim role, but not these patients.

Ottinger, Paul, and Jarvis and the Act of Confessing to One's Self

The other complicated aspect of understanding how gamblers use the act of medical confession is the act of self-persuasion (this refers to the discursive agent's relationship with self). Again, the act of self-persuasion is more complicated than it might at first sight appear. The self does not simply apply a unitary discourse to itself in a moment of self persuasion. Discourse must always find a way of fitting into a set of discourses already in place within the mind of the individual pathological gambler. In their negotiations with others, actors must also resolve their own internal difficulties regarding a particular discursive situation. At any given moment we are each a set of subtle, competing discursive perspectives that must fight out which discursive perspective will hold a relative position of dominance. We are each a concert of self. We are a concert of self melted outwardly inward into ourselves and society. We are a multi-singularity with no definite beginning or ending. We are a textual node that links to the beginning of discursive time; extending outward into the various fields of discursive relations making up our worlds. We intersect, inform one another, send discursive transmissions, connect with one another. Intersecting and interacting with information from everywhere within and without, we are in a constant state of reading—reading this, reading that, making sense, making meaning—with our being, our sense of self in relation to ourselves. Through this process we alter and shape the discursive web into which we are embedded. We arrange the discourses speeding through us, we give attention to certain texts over others; we ignore and place on back-up file old data and move to the front new. We are constantly shifting and altering, changing and accommodating. We are forever reorganizing the connecting points and the primary pathways of knowledge coming up from the deepest levels of collective and unconscious existence. In the process we push our alterations outward onto others, sharing the same and different texts, the links of communication buzzing. We are connected. We are playing the discursive game. We take it all mostly as real. We believe it to be true. It has consequences.

Take, for example, the pathological gambler. Most pathological gamblers never lose the desire to gamble. They have a certain set of pro-gambling discourses which are always in competition with the discourses of treatment. Comprised within these discourses are competing positions of morality, ways of caring for self, definitions of success and risk, ideas about the perceptions and opinions of others and so on. Like the devil and the angel on the opposite shoulders of a cartoon character, both trying to persuade the character in one direction or another, the discourses within the mind of the gambler compete to establish a position of control. The negotiations the gambler has with these discourses are dependent upon the situation taking place (e.g., is the gambler driving past a race track?), the institutional pressures the gambler is struggling with (e.g., the gambler fears gambling or the treatment staff has made it clear that continued gambling could result in death), and the social networks in which the gambler is embedded (e.g., is he around pro or anti-gambling friends or family?). All of these factors, the psychological and the social, intersect to form a dense web of discursive relations in which the beliefs and opinions of the actor are subject to change dependent upon what needs to be made known to get something done. This is the act of discursively negotiated self-persuasion.

If today the pathological gambler wants to gamble, then the medical model loses. If tomorrow the gambler wants to get his wife back, the medical model wins. It is this complicated process of socio-psychological, context-mind-discourse negotiations that helps us understand why actors relapse and return to treatment or why people do not behave consistent with their self-reports—people are always in flux, there is no clear boundary between person and context, actor and structure, written discourse and internal theories, and conceptualizations. The act of discursively negotiated self-persuasion is forever taking place, changing to fit the situation despite our habitual and often consistent attitudes, despite our perceptions and beliefs. We are always already more than the discourses within which we are embedded. There is no ultimate beginning or ending. It is only a matter of degree and position.

Chapter 11

THE WORLD OF INVETERATE GAMBLERS

The discourse of the winning inveterate gambler, the one who wins at gambling, the one who gambles because he or she not only loves to gamble but is good at it, is radically different from those inveterates who are within, be it for however long, the confines and negotiated thinking structures of the medical model—and accept, gladly or not, the label of pathological gambler as the primary discourse by which they define themselves. It is to the differences between the winners and the failures, therefore, that we must make a distinction.

To get a sense of the differences between the winning and losing inveterate gambler, we need to review two published statements by inveterate gamblers. In their differences they represent, as ideal types, the wider population of inveterate gamblers today and the major differences between those who seek treatment and those who do not. The first is by Bernie P., (Bernie P. and Bruns 1973) a self-diagnosed pathological gambler. Bernie P. is a failed gambler. The second is by John Bradshaw (1975), who wrote about gambling winners.

Bernie P. and the Failed Gambler

> Two gambling friends, Allen Klein and Joe Martin, shared my craving for Vegas, so when we pulled a $200,000 fur heist

(theft) in Montreal, it was only natural that we thought of escaping to but one place. What better town to turn our stolen $200,000 into $1,000,000 than Las Vegas. . . .

We swaggered into the Sands Hotel early Friday evening. . . . We checked into our room, took $25,000 out of our bags and headed down to the casino. . . . We headed straight for the crap table since dice was our favorite game. It was the fastest action, and you stood the best chance of running your stake into a fortune.

I started off betting $50 on the pass line, $50 on every box, and $50 behind the point—an average of $350 a roll. I held all the gambling money. We were a team and I was the real crap shooter. But right from the beginning I was a loser. Before long my bets were $100, then $200, then $300, and then the house limit—which amounted to $3,500 a roll. At first, all through Friday night, we had so much money that we didn't notice our losses. But the $200,000 steadily dribbled away—a thousand here, two thousand there. I would have lucky periods, but when I did I was just recouping the earlier losses. I could never get ahead. Yet I refused to leave the table. I was afraid the table might get hot just as I left . . . .

I gambled all through Saturday and into Saturday night, still at the same table, losing boldly, with only a few soaring moments to keep our plunge from showing. Joe and Allen wandered off to gamble on their own, but I went through every set of croupiers and, when the original crews began returning for the second time, they smiled at me knowingly. The cocktail waitress would bring me a sandwich or a cup of coffee and I would leave only to go to the bathroom. I truly was frightened that I might miss a hot period. I grabbed a couple of quick naps, but I made sure my friends stayed at the table to rush and wake me up if the dice got hot.

Early Sunday morning, about two a.m., we decided to meet back at the hotel room to count up our remaining money. There was $70,000 left. "Let's get out of town before we blow it all," argued Allen. But Joe and I wouldn't given in. "Our luck has to turn sometime," I said, trying to give my voice an edge of confidence. "Yeah," replied Joe, "we came here to give it our best shot. Let's stick it out through Sunday." Back we went downstairs, to the same table. By daybreak we had lost another $25,000 . . . . By mid-afternoon we were broke, flat busted.

When we got together in the lobby of The Sands, near a bank of slot machines, we counted up our money: one quarter and one dime. Thirty-five cents. We talked morosely about how we were going to get back to New York, but actually we all knew that was no problem, we could always forge some checks. We were stalling for an excuse to stay in town. I didn't even feel I was gambled out. As we sat there moaning about our bad luck, we watched an old lady playing a quarter slot machine. She fed the machine for nearly a half hour without hitting a jackpot. Finally, she walked away. I looked at my partners and they nodded towards the machine. "Okay," I said, "here goes." I got up, went over and fed the machine our last quarter. To my delight, twelve quarters came tumbling out. "Wow," said Joe, "now that's the kind of luck we need."

That gave us an idea . . . . We decided to sit around and watch for more people giving up on unproductive slot machines, then try our luck when the odds seemed best for a payoff. All we wanted to do, we thought, was scrape up enough money to pay our fares back to New York.

It took us about three hours but we were lucky enough at our little game and we managed to accumulate $60. We couldn't resist the casino inside, luring us with its flashing dice and shuffling chips. We split our money three ways . . . .

I got a lucky run of the dice, making my number six straight times and pretty soon we had run up our pile to almost $700. But we didn't leave . . . . I grinned and doubled my bets. "Damn, I told you our luck is changing!" I said. "I can just feel it!" The dice came to me and I pushed $200 out on the line and began rolling. I was back in action and I was hoping to win back that $200,000.

I worked my stake up to $4,300 before that table began cooling off. I decided to take a quick break to buy something I had always wanted to own. A pair of alligator shoes. I had been, in my own mind, a big-time gambler for fifteen years and yet I had never owned a pair of alligator shoes . . . . [At Sy Devore's]

I found a pair I liked, had them delivered to our room—using my pseudonym, Bernie Portnoy—and returned to the casino.

Joe and I hit a long cold spell and within an hour we had lost our money. After our last chips were pulled away by the croupier we remained at the table, unable to believe that once again we didn't have a dollar left between us . . . .

When Allen didn't return, we decided to go to the room and start to pack. At least he would have money to get us back to New York. I found the alligator shoes on the bed and put them on. I felt good. About an hour later he joined us.

"How'd you do?" he asked quickly. "We're busted," I said . . . . Allen was stunned. "We can't leave. I don't have a dime!" . . . In those days, being broke in Vegas was like being in the middle of the Sahara Desert without water.

Suddenly there was a knock on the door. "Come in," I shouted. And in walked the salesman from Sy Devore's, a tall thin fellow.

"Mr. Portnoy?" he asked. "I've come to collect $75."

"You got the wrong room, kid," growled Joe. But I interrupted, "No, that's the name I'm using."

"I'm sorry, Mr. Portnoy," the kid went on, "but I was sent to get the money."

"I'm tapioca," I said.

"I'm sorry about that, Mr. Portnoy." Then he kneeled down, pulled off my alligator shoes and put them in a box.

I watched in mournful silence as he walked out of the room, closing the door gently behind him. There I was, broke, two thousand miles from home, and sitting in my stocking feet." (Bernie P. and Bruns 1973, pp. 7–17)

John Bradshaw and the Winning Gambler

It began, I suppose, with the tales—the tales of gambling for immoderate sums at craps and cards, at pool, at golf and backgammon. The old gamblers would talk into the night, recalling the days when for a bet of twenty thousand Titanic Thompson pitched a key into its lock or when Nick the Greek, on his final card, filled an inside straight and won a half a million. . . . They liked to talk about the past and spoke of it in present tenses. . . . Despite their age they were hard, shrewd men and put aside my claims that they, perhaps, were merely sentimental. No, the times had changed, they said, the country had aged, become somehow tame and uniform. . . .

In the beginning, I had some indefinite plan to write an account of winners and losers and toward the end had come to Vegas in search of suitable candidates. But it soon became quite clear that while losers flourished everywhere, winners were a rare and reticent breed with preferences for camouflage and anonymity. Having talked to the bookmakers, the pit bosses, the shills, the dealers, the croupiers, all of whom professes intimate and accurate views of the matter, even then, a dark confusion continued to hobble through my mind. How could one be sure? What esoteric qualities actually separated a winner from a loser?

Taught from the start to believe in absolutes, I found myself still half in love with the lie that losers were unlucky, that winners were merely fortunate— privy to none of those sudden catastrophes that snap at the heels of lesser men. . . . Nick the Greek, possibly the most notorious of American gamblers, claimed that the only difference between winners and losers was one of character, which, he added, was about the only difference one could find between people anyway. But Nick held a rigid view of the world—heads or tails, win or lose, no two ways about it. He was a gambler and gamblers incline to unconditional views.

Understandably, it was the winner, the successful gambler, who came to intrigue me more and more. Seen in retrospect, there was a certain magic in their lives. They seemed somehow blessed to me, inhabiting some strange and utterly unknowable kingdom. Their casual command of dice and cards, of odds and probabilities, their puzzling immunity to lures of cash or high stacks of multicolored chips astonished me. And yet, when looked at logically—at play, in conversation—they appeared to be such ordinary men.

For more than a year, I consorted with six such men, not to define myself or them, but to understand that part of myself I believed we had in common . . . . In effect, I wished to know what kind of men they were, what is was like to win and win consistently.

To begin with, it would be helpful to explain what a winner is not. It has long been fashionable in psychiatric circles to refer to gamblers as flagrant examples of a particular kind of neurotic behavior. According to the late Dr. Edmund Bergler, all gamblers are, in varying degrees, compulsive losers. It is not therefore surprising that such groups as Gamblers Anonymous have used Bergler's text to reinforce their own contention that gambling is not only morally indefensible, but the outward symptoms of a diseased and crippled mind . . . . Such views, of course, tend to fall in line with the traditional moral attitudes toward gambling, particularly in America. That is, that the gambler is a low jade, remotely romantic perhaps, but intimate with all the usual vices. . . .

Thus, the classic description of the gambler has come to be defined not only as that of a born loser, but a compulsive loser as well. . . . But I am not concerned with them. I am more interested in a different species altogether—a small minority of men who are, if anything, compulsive winners. . . .

In the strictest sense, they are not even gamblers. . . . They are, in the best sense, gamesmen—experts at specific games.

Gambling, however, invariably involves a certain risk and the success or failure of that risk is rewarded or punished in terms of money. It is the greed and hence the fear of money that intoxicates most gamblers. With professionals, however, money is considered in another light and so acquires a different value . . . .

In those high-rolling circles of which I speak, money is a means of keeping score, nothing more. There is a case in point in the tale of the gambler who arrived at one of the larger Eastern tracks some years ago with five dollars in his pocket . . . . In the first race of the afternoon he bet five dollars on the second favorite and the horse came in paying $30. In the second race he bet the $30 on a long shot going off at 12-to-1. The horse won easily and the gambler collected $390. . . . By the sixth race, he had amassed $4,000 and he placed it all on the

> nose of a 3-to-1 shot. The horse, a tip from one of his friends in the paddock, spurted from behind to beat the favorite in a photo finish. The gambler now had $16,000 in his pocket. In the final race of the day he bet the lot on the heavy favorite [and the horse lost]. Buttoning his rumpled suit, he shuffled slowly from the track. At the main entrance he was hailed by an old acquaintance, who asked how he had fared that afternoon. Lighting a cigarette, the gambler shrugged and said, "Not bad, not bad. I lost five dollars" . . . .
>
> [I]t is beyond the imagination of a true conservative to comprehend a man who feels no special allegiance to money, a man who will risk all for the risk itself. Such men [gamblers] are confined to a special solitude of their own making. They are not prepared to pay the moral-social tax that society attempts to extract from the rest of us. They have no desire to do well, to get ahead, to set a good example and they remained, for the most part, undefeated. There was about them a superb and enviable insouciance. When they have gone, something important, some last fine flamboyant gesture will have vanished with them.
>
> These men shared that passion which someone once called the joyful acceptance of risk. Beyond that there was little they had in common. It was only in the pursuit of their passion that they could be said to have been alike. . . . They were excessive men and now and then overreached themselves; but these were trifling retrogressions. From the beginning, each of them believed that the force of passion would somehow see him through. Much later, when I first encountered them, these six men, the separate sons of a telephone repairmen, a bootlegger, a gambler, an oil executive, an evangelist, and a soldier of fortune, continued to believe with some queer unquenchable conviction that given time and talent and happy odds all things were possible. (Bradshaw 1975, pp. 1–8)

Reading the stories of Bernie P. and John Bradshaw, it is apparent that there is a difference between the inveterate gambling winner and the inveterate gambling failure. But what is the difference? Is it the losing itself—that is, their involvement in the chase, as described in chapter three—or is it in the way the gambler approaches the entire process of gambling?

To date, the most in-depth analysis of inveterate gamblers—and the differences between winning and losing gamblers—comes from the work of John Rosecrance (e.g., 1985b, 1986a, 1986b, 1989). John Rosecrance is a sociologist and a self-admitted inveterate gambler. His passion is horse racing. He has spent his life around the track and made gambling his professional work as well. Being both a sociologist and a gambler, Rosecrance's work is written from the perspective of the winning inveterate gambler, which is unique in the gambling literature. The field of gambling studies is primarily based on the clinical accounts of individuals already self-defined as pathological gamblers. Rosecrance's research is different. He gives the reader a first-hand account of gamblers "in action." But not just "in action" and losing. We get "in action" and winning.

Whether or not Rosecrance intended it this way, his work reads as an apologetic on behalf of winning inveterate gamblers. Throughout his work, whether he is attacking the medical model or offering alternative suggestions for treatment, he is always making a distinction between gambling winners and failures. According to Rosecrance, gambling failures are not representative of inveterate gamblers as a whole. Those that end up in treatment or spend a life-time in GA or the medical model are often a different type of person. And so, a distinction must be made.

First of all, what makes someone an inveterate gambler—whether they are a winner or not—is the approach they have to gambling itself. Simply put, inveterates love to gamble and so gambling is a way of life for them. Beyond that, what distinguishes the winners from the failures has to do with their approach to the losing phase itself. Winners understand how to handle losses and go on to gamble another day. They therefore spend the majority of their lives outside the confines of the medical model and its trappings. Gambling failures, however, do not. For one reason or another, inveterate gambling failures get caught up in the chase, and find themselves often falling out of gambling into the medical model, some staying within it for a short period of time, others for good.

Gambling Winners

So what about the winners? If winners don't suffer from psychological problems, then why do they like to gamble so much? The reason has to do with aesthetics and the ability to successfully care for oneself different from mainstream morality and our dominant socio-capitalistic conceptions of how one should live in relation to money and risk.

Bradshaw (1975) illustrated the world of the winner, the successful gambler, the gambler without addiction, without compulsion, without pathology. In the gambling world, Bradshaw's gamblers are heroes, living legends. They engage in a proper care of self. They have no concern for money in the manner of the capitalist. They have no concern for mainstream morality, or the mental hygiene prescribed by the medico-psychological discourses dominant in American society. They recoil against such confinement. They put off the American dream; they laugh at it. They have no concern for their case to be heard in the courtroom. They have no opinion of gambling legislature. They will gamble and gamble well, regardless what the dominant forms of government have to say. Their sense of a proper care of self does not come from the outside. It comes from within their own world. They are the masters of it. They have defined the rules, the codes, the aesthetics. Within their own world(s) they are winners.

Outside their worlds, however, as gambling becomes increasingly recognized as a medical problem, they are being forced to negotiate with everyone: family, friends, employers, government, business, GA, the councils, and so on. These negotiations come in the form of daily hassles with people over the way they live their lives. Family members disagree with their approach to money, their approach to work, the way they spend their time. Employers are suspicious of their heavy gambling activity. They are often hustled by the police, the courtroom, the various institutes of social control. And let us not forget the medical model.

As the medical model invades our cultural landscape, it ever so gently sneaks up the inveterate's back until doubts and questions begin to arise about the lifestyle they have chosen. When so many are opposed to a lifestyle, be it whatever, it is a constant battle to defend one's right to live as one so chooses. As the medical model moves in and labels all forms of excessive gambling as pathological, inveterates will have to rework their negotiations in order to ward off the power of treatment. The medical model, as it did with depression, anxiety, neurosis, and addiction, will slowly become, regardless of its various restraints through government and business and so on, part of the cultural vocabulary of the average United States citizen. As it increases in power, inveterates will be up against a whole new form of domination, normalization, surveillance, and control. And they will have to struggle to safeguard the ability to live freely and openly without having to defend constantly against the discourses of the medical model. These are the discursive negotiations of inveterates, the struggles they face as we approach the turn of the century.

Gambling Failures

According to Rosecrance (1986a, 1986b), of the various skills necessary to make it through the losing phase of gambling, two are the most important: perception and attribution. After experiencing a serious loss in gambling, which Rosecrance calls a "bad beat," it is very common for gamblers to chase their loses. The difference between the winners and the failures is how they deal with the losing phase: how they perceive losing and what they attribute as the cause. Winners, it seems, are able to recover from the loss to go on to win again; failures do not. Instead, they continue to purse their losses. Their reasons for pursuing these loses can be a result of problems with impulsivity, attention deficit disorder and so on. Nevertheless, it is when they become involved in the chase that they become susceptible to being labeled a pathological gambler.

Building upon Lesieur's (1977) notion of the chase, a person becomes a failure if they have gambled far too much money and get into trouble with the law, or, as Wedgeworth explains (1998), their financial losses and level of gambling create strained relationships with family members and friends, and can no longer defend their gambling. As a result, they, for the time being, fall out of the world of gambling. They are no longer able to maintain their lifestyle. For the moment, they are trapped within a deviant status. In our socio-capitalistic culture, what defines the difference between a winner and a failure, between a person who enters treatment and a person who doesn't, is whether or not they can recover quickly enough from their loses. If they can't recover quickly enough, then usually someone important to them, such as a family member, a law officer, an employer, a parent, a spouse, a child, will eventually define them as a gambling failure. At this point the outside person often challenges the gambler regarding his or her relative success. If labeled as a failure from the outside, the gambler, feeling estranged from his or her gambling lifestyle, may give in to the pressures of the *outsider* and accept the label.

At the point of failure, pathological gamblers have one of several options. Some escape the situation by leaving their family and friends to go somewhere else. Some find a new set of gamblers to hang out with. Others may find more money, do their jail time, or try to con their way out of their problems, or even stop gambling all together. After a short amount of time, however, most will return to gambling to start the process all over again. A small few even go on to be winners again. A good percentage, however, decide to enter treatment. Once they make this decision, they enter into the medical model. This, then, is the difference between the inveterate gambling winner and the gambling failure.

But, this leaves us with a question: if Rosecrance is so opposed to the medical model, what does he suggest we do with the inveterate gambling failure?

Teaching the Gambling Failures to Be Winners

Being true to form, Rosecrance (1986a, 1986b, 1989) argues that gambling failure is a function of misperception and attribution alone. What inveterates therefore need is a treatment program that teaches them how to be better gamblers; they need to be taught controlled gambling.

Rosecrance outlines his ideas for a controlled gambling treatment program in his 1989 article "Controlled Gambling: A Promising Future." He has four major ideas for treatment, which are based on the research of David Oldman (1978). Oldman explained that the most important message people with pathological gambling and those who treat them need to hear is that "this particular mechanism whereby one reaches a crisis point is a consequence not of personality defect but of a defective relationship between strategy of play on the one hand and a way of managing one's finances on the other" (pp. 369–370).

Building on Oldman, Rosecrance makes four suggestions for treatment. First, gamblers should be taught more appropriate gaming strategies and money management (1989, p. 152). Second, therapists should learn to have more empathy for gamblers who want to maintain some form of sustained gambling (p. 152). Third, both gamblers and therapists need to understand that most of the gambler's ineffective coping strategies are manifested outside of the counseling setting (p. 152). And fourth, therapists and gamblers need to bring into treatment "winning" gamblers to help teach more appropriate gambling strategies (p. 152).

Putting these four basic aspects of treatment into practice, the style of treatment itself would be based largely on peer counseling, and a *controlled-gambling* treatment plan. The combination of these two aspects of treatment would help to produce an individual who no longer gambles in an out of control manner. The actor would have a greater level of control, and therefore would not fall into all of the psychological and social problems that are so often associated with gambling, including crime. This could be the answer to the middle-class creation of gambling as a new social problem. Instead of misdirecting these individuals into in-patient medical treatment programs or sending them to jail over and over again, we would teach them how to be winners.

To validate the potential success of this alternative approach to treatment, Rosecrance provided the results of an in-depth study he did on fifty gamblers who completed treatment at Sartin Clinic for Controlled Gambling in Southern California. These inveterates "had lost businesses, homes, spouses, and financial resources all to gambling. Some had served time in jails or prisons for gambling-related thefts. Several had attended Gamblers Anonymous meetings. [In short,] no one could deny they had been 'true' problem gamblers. However, after changing their betting strategies and money managing practices . . . most had been able to overcome their problem gambling, and were now managing participation in an acceptable manner. Not all had become winning gamblers . . . but they were able to keep losses within manageable parameters" (1989, p. 157).

Rosecrance and the Cognitive-Behaviorists

While not gamblers themselves—and therefore, not direct representatives of the experiences of inveterates—other treatment experts have been in support of Rosecrance's conceptualization of failed inveterate gamblers. Those most strongly in support of his ideas have been the cognitive-behaviorists.

The primary goal of the cognitive-behaviorists has been to challenge the medical model to include a *dimensional approach* to gambling addiction. The dimensional model argues that "pathological gambling is an end point on a continuum that ranges from no gambling through to heavy and problematic gambling and that social learning principles are important determinants of an individual's position on that continuum at any given time" (Blaszczynski and McConaghy 1989, p. 43). Therefore, while cognitive-behaviorists attend to biological and physiological processes, they primarily focus on therapeutic techniques that emphasize the role of environment and learning, such as bio-feedback, behavior modification, and systematic desensitization (e.g., Blaszczynski and Silove 1995; Dickerson and Weeks 1979; Roby 1995).

The theorists comprising this position are represented by Blaszczynski (1985), McConaghy (1991), Blaszczynski and McConaghy (1989), Blaszczynski and Silove (1995), Blaszczynski, McConaghy and Frankova (1991), Dickerson (1979, 1984, 1993), Dickerson and Weeks (1979) and Roby (1995). Of the various authors, the most recognized is Blaszczynski, who is a clinical psychologist from Australia. His analyses of controlled gambling were done at The Prince of Wales Hospital in Randwick, Australia. Because of his support of the dimensional model of pathological gambling, Blaszczynski and his colleagues hold four important positions in contrast to the medical model of pathological gambling.

First, they do not believe that gambling is necessarily a progressive and chronic illness (Blaszczynski and McConaghy 1989; Dickerson 1984). From a dimensional model perspective, while the continued inability to control one's losses will lead, as Lesieur would argue, to inevitable destruction, this does not mean that these behaviors are immune to change. It is not, as GA would say, that "pathological gambling is a progressive illness which can be arrested but never cured" (Gamblers Anonymous 1984). Cognitive-behaviorists believe that excessive gambling is the result of ineffective coping skills, problems with impulsivity, misperceptions of one's environment, and poor gambling strategies. All of these problems can be cured by good therapy and training. While an excessive gambler can progress in his losses, so can a business that lacks effective fiscal strategies and a good accountant or two. And you certainly wouldn't say that a failed business suffers from a disease.

Second, cognitive-behaviorists do not rigidly adhere to the narrow definition of gambling provided by the DSM. Because there is no one reason why excessive gamblers lose control, and because the consequences of gambling can vary in both degree and style, it is impossible to reduce the problems of excessive gambling to a medical diagnosis alone. To do so is to remove the phenomena from its context. Blaszczynski and McConaghy (1989) state: "No single characteristic appears to differentiate pathological from nonpathological gamblers. Characteristics such as incapacity to stop, hedonistic abandonment, psychological need to lose or neurosis would appear to be products of post-hoc value-laden judgement" (p. 46).

Third, as the quote above reveals, because of their arguments against the DSM and the "progression" model of gambling, cognitive-behaviorists fail to see a clear and distinct difference in psychological profile or gambling behavior between regular and excessive gamblers. Blaszczynski and McConaghy (1989) state: "Proponents of the dimensional model argue that there is as yet no empirical evidence available to support the claim that pathological gamblers form a categorical group distinct from social gamblers" (p. 44–45). It is pointless to continue onward in the literature to reify the DSM and make the affirmation of the gambling diagnosis the beginning and end of any study. Research done in support of Blaszczynski and McConaghy's argument includes Oldman (1978) and Dickerson (1984).

Of the various positions held by the cognitive-behaviorists, the most important is their shared belief with Rosecrance that controlled gambling is a viable option for treatment. Abstinence is not always necessary nor realistic. If pathological gambling is a failure in learning, and not a disease in the strict sense of the word, then it makes sense that once taught to control themselves, gamblers could return to a more stable gambling lifestyle. This is the premise that has guided the research in controlled gambling. In a study to compare the self-reported level of mental and emotional health in pathological gamblers two to nine years post-treatment, Blaszczynski, McConaghy, and Frankova (1991) found that those gamblers who had control over their gambling, be it through complete or partial abstinence, were healthier emotionally, psychologically, and relationally, than those without control. They therefore concluded that while total abstinence is still recommended, it is not always necessary: "Although the findings of this study suggested controlled gambling is an acceptable outcome, it seems prudent to encourage abstinence as the preferred treatment goal until predictor variables are available which could identify the subjects able to maintain controlled gambling following treatment" (p. 305).

The Marginalization of Rosecrance and the Cognitive-Behaviorists

If the dimensional model of pathological gambling provides a broader and more sophisticated conceptual and theoretical framework for understanding and treating pathological gambling, then why is the medical model still in a position of relative dominance? It seem that while theoretically strong, the ideas of Rosecrance and the cognitive-behaviorists presents too great a political, professional, and economic challenge to medicine and addiction treatment. For those readers who are in the field of addiction, you know that to mention *controlled* gambling, drinking, or drug usage as a viable treatment alternative is, as Coleridge states, to wear the albatross around one's neck. It is certain professional death. Not to mention writing articles in direct disagreement with either the medical model or the disease conception of gambling, as Blaszczynski (1985) has. In a society such as ours where the *war on drugs* is seen by many (along with poverty) as our most important battle, *controlled usage* is close to heresy. If addiction counselors started arguing that controlled usage is a more viable way to define treatment outcome and recovery, what would be the basis for continuing the war on drugs? Our entire national "medical" rhetoric would have to change. As Blaszczynski and McConaghy (1989) explain, this is unlikely to happen: "Disappointingly, the literature to date contains only one controlled outcome study in which two differing behavioral techniques were compared. Although research in general has focused on identifying the nature of cognitive distortion in gambling, findings for these studies have not been systematically translated into treatment programs" (p. 195).

And so, as we progress through the 1990s, winning inveterate gamblers and their alternative lifestyles remain under attack and are too easily swept in with the gambling failures. If Rosecrance is to be given any credit, the challenge researchers and clinicians must face as they approach the next century is to make the distinction between those who do and do not need treatment, and to make sure that the distinction is not based on a love of gambling itself, but on the spectrum of problems which make the chase an addictive and devastating process for some people and not for others.

Chapter 12

THE FAMILY: A GROUP WITH NO DISCURSIVE VOICE

At Torniero's pre-trial hearing, everyone was well represented. Even the pathological gamblers and inveterates who didn't have a voice at least had someone there on their behalf. The medical experts had their guns: the fields of gambling research and treatment, Gamblers Anonymous, and the Gambling Councils. The gambling industry, criminal justice system and government had their supporters as well. In terms of experts, the trial was well represented—well represented that is, except for one decidedly omitted voice, the families.

One of the most remarkable aspects of Torniero's pre-trial hearing was that none of the major issues being discussed—responsibility and rights, punishment and rehabilitation—were addressed in terms of their impact on the family members and friends of pathological gamblers. During the entire trial, not once did either the defense or prosecution raise this as an issue or question. In fact, throughout the 1980s and 1990s, while the debates over the medical model raged on, little to no attention was given to the family members. This happened because, while not necessarily intended, the concerns of the family for the past eighteen years have consistently fallen outside the purview of all the major discourses devoted to this issue—from government and the gambling industry to the criminal justice system and the medical model. The goal of this chapter is to review how and why.

Government

The first and most obvious reason why families have been ignored has been because of our government's silence on the issue. While the government has said very little about pathological gambling in general, it has said even less about an issue that is yet another manifestation of domestic violence and family breakdown. Pathological gamblers are often physically and mentally abusive to their spouses and family members (Berman and Siegel (1992). They neglect their responsibilities at home, lie to family and friends, become addicted to alcohol and drugs, empty their bank accounts, leave their parents with unpayable debt, and ignore and victimize their kids. They are consistently unable to take responsibility for their actions. And so, the family picks up the slack. In fact, wherever a pathological gambler is, there you will find a small group of dysfunctional devotees. If the gambler has no one else around, the gambler is surely on her last leg.

The girlfriends, the boyfriends, the parents, and the children all pay a price for their relationships with the pathological gambler. Their time, their money, their desires, and their lives are all sacrificed. As the pathological gambler falls further into the chase, everyone around him slowly becomes an object for his usage. A child or wife is no longer a human being to be embraced and cared for. To find love, to find compassion, family and friends must often decide to live their lives in relation to the pathological gambler. Everything else ends up being sacrificed—moved to the background, warped, broken, fractured, ignored.

Unfortunately, because government remains silent and doesn't engage in a "war" on this issue, family and friends fail to see the power they have to change their lives. They fail to see their ability to construct an independent voice, a voice that would otherwise tell them to escape their private hell. And so their voice becomes only an echo in the back of their mind. Sometimes it rushes to the surface, screams out for attention. But it is quickly silenced, shut back down, forced to take a subservient position. So strong are the effects of pathological gambling that even years after they've left the gambler, or the gambler has stopped gambling, family and friends continue to work through the process of healing. This reality becomes even more troubling given the fact that most pathological gamblers are still men—which means that the health of women is once again being ignored:

> She tried to remember. When had it begun? How long had it taken to reach this point? When was it he had become preoccupied with watching football games on television? When had it become a sacrosanct happening that nobody dared disturb without being subjected to an abusive, intemperate scolding? When was it they had started to quarrel about his gambling, and then about other things that had nothing to do with gambling, things about which they had never quarreled before? When was it he had started to react with explosions of elation after some games and spells of dejection, lasting for days, after others? . . .
>
> Friends had asked her, after the marriage was over, how she could have continued to live in that hell for so long without fleeing, without going out of her mind. Why had it taken her so long to free herself of this life of torture and misery? And she had remained quiet, pretending she did not know the answer, not wanting to relive the pain. How could they know what it meant to be caught in a maelstrom, whirled about and pinned down by powerful, paralyzing forces, unable to generate enough counterforce to move even an inch, let alone to break out of its control? . . . It took everything she had in emotional strength just to cope with each episode and get over it, to survive just for that day. . . .
>
> How had all of this come about and why? What had happened to this man? What was it that made him change? . . . She put her hands to her temples and squeezed, trying to shut off this train of thought, the painful memories, the insistent questions to which she could find no answers. (Custer and Milt 1985 pp. 7–9)

The Gambling Industry

Despite how much noise the gambling industry has made about pathological gambling, they've given no attention to the problems of the family. They've given no attention to the problems of the family because their troubles are meaningless; meaningless, that is, as long as they pay their loved one's debt. It will be interesting to see what happens once families start suing casinos and horse tracks on a more regular basis for the debts incurred by their loved ones. Only then will the gambling industry start to take notice of this problem. Only then will the issues of responsibility and right, punishment and rehabilitation, extend to address the concerns of the family.

At the present moment, however, as pointed out by Rose (1988), the gambling industry has chosen to ignore the problem. He states: "Direct and indirect harm to the gambler and his family, including suicide, divorce, loss of jobs and imprisonment are the greatest threat to the legal industry; and yet, it is the one area where the industry is doing surprisingly little. Newspapers regularly report damage awards in the millions of dollars, and yet the casinos, race tracks and lotteries of America have taken few steps to protect their clientele from themselves" (p. 257). To further back his point, Rose (1988) cites the case of Wynn v. Monterey Club, in which the defendant—the husband of a pathological gambler—sued the Monterey Club casino because they gave his wife check cashing privileges even though he had explicitly told them not to. The case was thrown out of court, but it did set a precedent: in the future, the voices of the family will have to be heard; their suffering cannot continue to go unnoticed. Read the words of yet another story:

> The fun of gambling came to an end about the time our son entered junior high school. My husband's drinking increased with his gambling. It soon seemed to me that Peter was spending more of his free time in the bar, where he could place bets and then watch the games on which we'd wagered.
>
> Many times he would come home drunk and abusive. If he was drunk and had lost money, he would often become violent. At first he took out his anger on our belongings, then he got rough with me. As crazy as it may seem, I defended him to the children when they got angry at him for abusing me. Our children were very bright; they could see their father's anger coming from the alcohol in him and from the fact that he lost money gambling. . . .
>
> One time I threatened to leave Peter if he didn't stop gambling, because we couldn't pay our bills and our children were lacking necessities; I lacked everything. But I never left; instead, I got a part-time job. I wanted to pay off some of the

> bills, but the money I made wasn't enough, so in less than four months, I was working full time. It didn't take long to realize my working did only one thing—it gave him an opportunity to gamble more because I began taking on the responsibility of paying most of our family's expenses. I hardly ever noticed it happening. Peter was so manipulative and controlling, he got me to do that in no time at all. He even got me to feel that his gambling was my fault. I knew that was not true, but somehow I believed him. (Heineman 1992, pp. 53–54)

The Criminal Justice System

While, as we've seen throughout this study, the criminal justice system has dealt with a number of important issues concerning pathological gambling (see Rose 1988), they've yet to address the effect pathological gambling has on the family. A perfect example of this is the changing opinion judges have on the relevance of pathological gambling in divorce trials.

Rose (1988) states: "Now that compulsive gambling is gaining acceptance as a mental disorder outside of the individual's control, the law is becoming more lenient in its treatment of compulsive gamblers involved in divorce proceedings" (p. 252). This is great for pathological gamblers, but what about their spouses? What about the damage they've incurred? When do they get a break? When will someone understand their pain? The court's recognition of pathological gambling is an extremely important step forward. But, to make accommodations for this disorder without also taking into account the struggles of the family is to add insult to injury. Pathological gamblers can now not only cause undue pain and suffering to their spouses, they can also turn around and get out of what otherwise might have been a fair divorce or civil suit.

This lack of balance in perspective is a direct function of the unintentional negotiated interactions that have taken place between the medical model and the law over the past eighteen years. Because of the reductionistic approach of the medical model, when in court, the wider dimensions of the problem are not addressed. And so, as judges across the country make decisions about the relevance of pathological gambling to the practice of law, they do so without a full understanding of its impact on the family. As a result, the family is further marginalized and misunderstood:

> The police came shortly after midnight and rang and knocked and woke her up. Looking down from her bedroom window she saw the patrol car at the sidewalk, its lights flashing, and felt a surge of panic.
>
> When she came to the door, there were two of them standing there. One asked: "Are you __________?" And when she answered, "Yes," he said, "We have a warrant for your husband's arrest."
>
> "He doesn't live here. We were separated nine months ago."
>
> "We understand that he's been staying here."
>
> "He was here for a few days, but not for the past week."
>
> "How come he's been staying here if you're separated? Are you living together again?"
>
> She wanted to protest their intrusion into her private life, their arrogance. But there wasn't enough energy left for that. She had enough resentment, enough quarreling, enough confrontation and screaming, enough agitation and hatred to last her for the rest of her life and to leave some over for eternity. Now all she wanted was to be left alone, to not feel anything, to stay numb inside herself, to get through each day quietly, without incident, without hearing the telephone ring, without the stab of fear every time it did ring, without the insults and threats at the other end, without having to discuss the past with anybody. But here were the police asking questions, and the questions had to be answered.
>
> "No, we are not living together again."
>
> "Then why is he coming here?"
>
> "He isn't coming here; I told you it's been a week."
>
> "What about before then?"
>
> "He came here about 10 days ago . . . it was late at night. He said he had no place to sleep. He looked sick. I couldn't turn him away. So I told him he could sleep on the couch, but he would have to leave in the morning."
>
> "Then what happened after that?"

> "In the morning I gave him money to get a room at the Y and to get himself something to eat. I gave him enough for a week. Two days later he came back. He didn't go to the Y. He gambled the money and lost it. He's a compulsive gambler."
>
> She waited for a change of expression on their faces, some indication that these words—compulsive gambler—had some meaning for them, that they would understand now what she had lived through, that they would know that the person they were hunting was the victim of an obsession, that he could not help what he did. She hoped they might show a little sympathy. But nothing. Not a sign of acknowledgment. Not a flicker of compassion. The phrase "compulsive gambler" meant absolutely nothing to them. Or, if it did, they didn't care. (Custer and Milt 1985, pp. 1–2, italics mine)

The Medical Model

During the past eighteen years, the only discourse available to the family has been the medical model. Because it was the only discourse available, it deserves to be congratulated. But, we cannot extend this congratulations too far. The medical model has far too many short-comings to remain the only discourse available. It is important, therefore, to be critical so that we can understand how and why things need to change. The limitations of the medical model are three.

First of all, as we reviewed in chapter five, because addiction treatment is structured to care for one individual at a time and has as its primary focus the individual pathological gambler, the family is largely ignored during the treatment process. To their credit, some gambling treatment facilities do discuss family issues with gamblers and even, on occasion, bring in family for a session or two of family therapy. But, the family is always seen in relation to the gambler. Questions revolve around what the family is going to do once treatment comes to an end. If the family wants treatment, they are advised to seek their own counseling.

The second problem with gambling treatment is the timing. Most gamblers do not seek treatment until they are in a lot of trouble. By then the family has suffered a great deal. As a result, seldom do interventions come for the family early on when treatment is really needed. If we had a model of pathological gambling that embraced the entire family, then treatment would be provided whether or not the gambler wanted to stop gambling.

Finally, because of the medical model's narrow view, unless the family members of a pathological gambler are brought into treatment, their knowledge about pathological gambling comes from the gambler her or himself. As I explained earlier, Wedgeworth (1998) has shown that most gamblers seek treatment to fix their strained relationships. Once in treatment, it doesn't take much for these gamblers to realize that they can use the medical model to their advantage. These gamblers are not therapists. They want their family and friends on their side. They want them to be caring and understanding, not working through their own anger, depression or guilt. But, because most families have their own issues to work through, they're often insensitive to the gambler, tired of yet once again having to put the gambler's emotions before their own. The family needs the type of "systems therapy" help that the medical model doesn't provide. Therefore, at present, the only chance most family members have is GamAnon—which is a self-help group for the families and friends of pathological gamblers. But, even GamAnon is limited because these groups often are not available because so few of them exist. And so life goes on:

> As the years went by, I was always tired, sometimes to the point of exhaustion. The house was a mess and I couldn't even seem to make minor decisions. It might be two o'clock before I even thought of making the beds, and the laundry would pile up until William and the kids didn't have any socks left. Sometimes I would stand staring at my closet deciding what to wear; I couldn't decide what to watch on television and would walk around the supermarket in a daze, not knowing what cereal to buy. . . .
>
> The children seemed to feel the tension in the house. When Bill was fifteen he got into trouble with gambling at school. Later I learned that when the principal said he would call his parents, Bill begged him to just call his father, saying, "My Mom's not been well lately. Her back and all, and she just can't take the stress." So the principal called William, who came in and "smoothed things over" and never told me. I found out about it a year later when Bill was expelled for selling pot at school.

Anna was like my best friend instead of a daughter. It used to kill me the way William would dote on her one minute, and then later ignore her. But Anna seemed to take it all in stride. At least I thought so. Then when she was about nine things changed. She began to get into trouble at school for pushing other kids and, later, for stealing a pencil case from another child. I was constantly being called by the school, but I couldn't believe she did all those things at school because at home she was so good.

Anna is sixteen now and she's as good at school as she is at home. She's always at a friend's house—Faith's or Brenda's. But when she is home she helps me, and is always trying to smooth things out between William, Bill, and me. But sometimes she says that if I was more understanding of William, lost weight, and got some interests of my own he wouldn't gamble so much.

Bill is hard to take lately. He's twenty-one and he works for a printer in St. Louis. He's got a good job, but he gambles and drinks too much. I don't seem to have much luck with the men in my life. (Berman and Siegel 1992, pp. 113–114)

Chapter 13

THE JUDGE'S DECISION

Bringing the Study to a Close

Now that we've arrived at end of this study, it's time to come full circle to where we started: the 1983 pre-trial hearing of John Torniero. Throughout our study, Torniero's pre-trial hearing has been an epicenter for the expanding discursive negotiations occurring in the field of pathological gambling over the last eighteen years—as have the arguments raised by the prosecution and defense. The prosecution and defense have represented the two major views people have taken toward pathological gambling since the 1980 publication of the DSM-III. On one side there's the pro-medical model view, which has been supported by pathological gamblers, the fields of gambling research and treatment, Gamblers Anonymous, and the state and federal gambling councils. On the other side, there's the anti-medical model view, which has been supported by the gambling industry, government, the criminal justice system and inveterate gamblers. In the middle, somewhere, unsure exactly what to believe, has been the family.

In many ways, then, Torniero's pre-trial hearing has also acted as a window into how we, in contemporary society, deal with social problems. It is as Rose (1988) stated: "Law trails society. Changes occurring in the social order in America inevitably lead to conflicts and eventually to changes in the law. The changes that are taking place in contemporary society in the way we view gambling gives us a unique opportunity to observe this slow and painful process at work. The most dramatic confrontations between the old and the new are being fought out to determine basic notions of justice, punishment, and responsibility" (p. 257). And so, what conclusions have we reached?

The Judge's Decision

With both sides having completed the presentation of their arguments, it was time for Judge José A. Cabranes to make a decision. The negotiations were over. Cabranes decided in favor of the prosecution. He declared that pathological gambling was not severe enough a mental disorder to meet the standards established by the ALI test and that pathological gambling was not an adequate basis for Torniero's criminal behavior. In his court report on the pre-trial hearing, Cabranes had this to say:

> Accordingly, the court concludes that it is appropriate to exclude any expert evidence concerning the defendant's alleged 'compulsive gambling disorder.' The court nonetheless holds, for reasons spelled out below, that the full scope of the relief sought by the Government—abolition of the insanity defense—cannot be granted, in part because most of the relief sought can be afforded the Government on more narrow grounds. Thus, the court will grant the Government the limitation upon the defendant's evidence and instructions to the jury that it seeks in this case. While today's ruling pertains specifically to today's case, the court is not unaware of other cases and of the social and legal climate within which the instant case arises. It shares the widespread and growing public concern that new mental disorders appear to be fabricated in unending succession, that psychiatrists often are required to submit themselves to public grilling by skilled advocates, and that defendants increasingly seek to 'explain' their alleged criminal acts as somehow compelled by pathologies of vague description and scant relevance. For more than a century, the insanity defense has expanded its role in our criminal justice processes. Today, the court declines the Government's invitation to 'abolish' that defense. The court does, however, hold that the defense can and should be limited

> to instances where a jury could find that the defendant's mind was truly alienated from ordinary human experience at the time of the commission of the acts with which he is charged and where that mental condition had a direct bearing on the commission of those acts. (United States v. Torniero 570 F. Supp 721. 1983. pp. 723–724)

Cabranes was not alone in his opinion. After four days of testimony, it took the jury at Torniero's criminal trial less than one hour to deliberate. They found Torniero guilty on eight of the ten counts he was charged with. Torniero served a "three-year prison term, to be followed by five years' probation and an ongoing duty to pay restitution to his victims. The trial judge also recommended that Torniero undergo treatment for his compulsive gambling affliction" (United States v. Torniero 735 F.2d 725. 1984. p. 728). Following the criminal trial, defense attorney Keefe appealed the decision. The appellate court ruled in favor of the prosecution and upheld the criminal court's decision. The case was closed.

And So What Have We Learned?

In 1848, the prescient, Prussian pathologist Virchow wrote that in our Modern era: "Medicine is a social science, and politics nothing but medicine on a grand scale." (Gerhardt 1989, p. 272). In our study of the history of pathological gambling, these words have rung true. Throughout the eighteen years that the medical model has been negotiated in and between the various positions comprising the field of pathological gambling—from the gambling industry and government to the field of inpatient treatment and the criminal justice system—a variety of interesting outcomes have occurred (such as the merger between the gambling industry and field of gambling treatment, and the merger between state gambling councils and government). But, these negotiations are far from over. The medical model, while it has made its impact, has only begun to influence the field of pathological gambling. The future holds many more discursive negotiations.

And so, what have we learned from these stories—this history of pathological gambling? Hopefully, we've learned that our current understanding of pathological gambling is not a function of research and clinical investigation alone. There are individual, political, institutional, professional, and economic factors involved as well. Understanding how these "non-clinical" and "non-empirical" factors influence the way we think about pathological gambling is important because it has serious repercussions for the way we care for ourselves and others. Lives hang in the balance. It is necessary that we do something.

PART III

Chapter 14

EPILOGUE: ADDRESSING THE PROBLEMS OF PATHOLOGICAL GAMBLING

In many ways, our tour through the history of the medicalization of pathological gambling has raised as many questions as it has answered—the most important being: if not the medical model, then what? My goal in this chapter is to provide one possible solution to this question by outlining a number of important changes that I believe need to take place if we are to move beyond our current limitations in thinking about and caring for this important social problem.

Rewriting the Medical Model

1. *We need to replace the medical model of pathological gambling with a bio-psycho-social discursive framework.* In a lot of ways, the field of gambling studies' marginalization from the larger social sciences has been a blessing in disguise. It's been a blessing in that conferences are small and often attended equally by researchers, clinicians, council members, representatives from the gambling industry and people in recovery. We should capitalize on such a high level of inter-action and construct an overarching theoretical framework that brings all of these various perspectives together. In fact, at one of the next national conferences, a session should be put together where people can come and brainstorm on a framework that would

be not only bio-psycho-social in emphasis, but politically, economically, historically, and culturally astute to the needs of all people involved.

2. *We need discourses that continue to challenge the authority, position, and power of the medical model.* The idea here is to figure out ways to make the best of the medical model while escaping its reductionistic clutches. Researchers can do this by taking time to integrate their ideas into a broader bio-psycho-social framework. Again, such a theory is needed first, but it would not take long to construct. Researchers can also guard against the media by taking time to clarify the limited generalizability of any one study and the need to think about the problems of pathological gambling from a more exhaustive perspective. Clinicians should do the same. Patients and their families should be educated to the political context of the disease concept. Pathological gamblers should be taught just what this concept means—and the clinical strengths and weaknesses so derived. Council members and GA can follow suit by likewise adopting a bio-psycho-social framework. The National Council has done this, for example, by putting its emphasis on problem, rather than just pathological, gambling. The new name conveys a broader agenda. And, lastly, by putting into practice a bio-psycho-social framework, we can challenge the gambling industry and government to see the growing field of gambling studies and treatment as more than just medicine. The binary oppositions between punishment and rehabilitation, and rights and responsibilities would no longer apply to our field, and so we would move on.

3. *We need to refrain from the urge to reduce pathological gambling to an issue of genetics and biochemistry.* We live in the age of the brain. Everything is being reduced to genetics and biochemical makeup—from criminal behavior to lifestyle preferences. We need to be careful of such popular thinking. Most geneticists are fully aware of the limitations of their findings. Popular culture, including the field of gambling treatment and research, often is not. Genetics is not the basis for pathological gambling. It is only one of a spectrum of contributing factors. We need to remember this point when making decisions about the importance of this area of study.

Treatment

Let us make no mistake, pathological gamblers *do* need treatment. I think pathological gambling is a serious disorder that requires treatment. Given my solid belief in the potential power of well constructed treatment, I make the following suggestions.

1. *We need to make treatment available.* Currently, very few "explicit" pathological gambling treatment programs exist in the United States. There is an easy solution to this problem. First, what we need to do is get our already existing addiction treatment facilities and mental health centers to extend their services to include pathological gambling. If addiction staff are educated to the similarities and differences between pathological gambling and other addictions, as well as taught the different therapeutic approaches that are useful, then pathological gamblers everywhere could receive the treatment they need—this would be particularly useful given the comorbidity of pathological gambling with other addictions and mental disorders. It would also be important to establish several leading treatment centers specifically devoted to the treatment of pathological gambling so they could lead the way in research and treatment.

2. *Treatment needs to be expanded to include families.* If pathological gambling is an addiction claiming roughly 3 percent of the population, this percentage, at the very least, doubles when you take into account the families. The impact pathological gambling has on the family needs to become an important and necessary part of treatment so that even if the pathological gambler is not interested in changing, the family still receives treatment.

There are already treatment professionals in the field of gambling studies dealing with this issue. Turning to these experts, we need to make available several conference seminars devoted to how family therapy can be integrated into existing treatment structures.

3. *While abstinence is a worthy goal for some pathological gamblers, it is not the best solution for everyone.* For a large percentage of the pathological and problem gambling population, controlled gambling is a viable option for treatment and a good way to measure the relative success of psychological and medical intervention (e.g., Blaszczynski, McConaghy, and Frankova 1991; Sharpe and Tarrier 1995; and Rosecrance 1988, 1989). If we continue to make abstinence our only goal, we short-change ourselves and our patients of the relative level of success possible through treatment. Despite the best treatment, pathological gamblers are going to do what they ultimately want. If we can teach them to at least have a greater sense of control over their lives—which the literature shows to be the most important factor to recovery—then we have taken important steps toward dealing with this problem.

4. *Treatment professionals need to educate the general population about the effects pathological gambling is having on the elderly populations and teenagers.* In states like Florida, pathological gambling amongst the elderly is rampant, and in states like Louisiana, adolescent gambling is as high as 8 percent. Treatment and education in the school systems and retirement communities is needed for this issue. For more information on the problems of the elderly community, contact the Florida Council on Compulsive Gambling (1-800-426-7711, nationwide). For more information on teenage gambling, see Mark Griffiths' (1995) *Adolescent Gambling.*

5. *Despite the therapeutic approach used, pathological gamblers have to take a certain amount of responsibility for their problems.* While pathological gambling is an addiction, gamblers must be taught to take responsibility for their past and present behavior. Most therapists do this already, but more emphasis should be placed on curbing the limits by which treatment can be used for purposes other than what it is intended for.

6. *We need to re-conceptualize the structure of in-patient gambling treatment.* If pathological gambling is a bio-psycho-social problem, then treatment needs to approach it as such. More emphasis needs to be placed on the social contexts to which patients return. If, for example, your population is largely working or middle-class males, you need to address problems of job dissatisfaction, boredom, economic recession, financial stability, gender role strain, marital and family relations, community support, and gambling availability. To neglect these issues is to set patients up for relapse. One way to deal with these problems is to establish a team approach to treatment, where psychiatrists, social workers, and community outreach professionals all work together. While this type of treatment costs more up front, it saves money in the long run. You do this by 1) making outreach available to patients at those critical moments, such as three, six, twelve and twenty-four months post-treatment, 2) focusing on controlled gambling rather than abstinence, 3) involving the entire family in treatment, and 4) involving community leaders, churches, and employers.

7. *HMO's and third-party insurance need to make it possible for pathological gamblers and their families to receive therapy.* Research and treatment outcome data need to be made available to insurance companies and HMOs. If these companies aren't aware of the seriousness of the problem, they don't understand why they need to make treatment available.

8. *Treatment professionals need to be given credit for their hard work.* Most professionals treating pathological gambling today do so with

strained budgets and limited resources. The hard work of these people needs to be recognized and congratulated.

9. *In treatment, we cannot reduce the problems of pathological gambling to the level of the individual.* The growing trend in health care today is to think of patient care in the aggregate. Gone are the days of treating one patient at a time. Treatment professionals can move to the cutting-edge of these changes by thinking of patient care in terms of diagnostic categories. For example, what is the success rate of your treatment program for those patients with attention deficit disorder, versus Axis-II disorders, versus clinical depression? Do you adjust your treatment plan accordingly to deal with these different sub-populations? Or what about differences in treatment for skilled versus luck gamblers? Or males or females; old versus young? The more sophisticated your program is to these differences, the more successful it will be in helping patients and gaining third-party payment support.

Diagnosis

1. *While the DSM-IV is useful, a more dynamic nomenclature is necessary.* The literature does not support the idea that pathological gamblers are a homogeneous population, and yet we continue to diagnose as if this were the case. There is no one type of pathological gambler. Instead, pathological gambling is the general behavioral manifestation of a variety of other problems—such as attention deficit, loss of identity, personality disorder, depression, failure at job, marital problems—as they play themselves out in the chase. Because diagnosis is essential to treatment, as well as a common vocabulary, our need to diagnosis at the level of behavior alone blinds us to the diversity of the patients we treat.

We can overcome this problem in two important ways. First, we leave the DSM diagnosis as is, only fixing it to better identify the behavioral dimensions of pathological gambling—such as, how the behavior of elderly pathological gamblers differs from the behavior of the young, and so on. Second, we construct a secondary diagnostic nomenclature that focuses on etiological differences. This secondary diagnostic system wouldn't be used to make the initial diagnosis, but would be used once the pathological gambler was identified. Questions for this second nomenclature would include such things as: 1) Do you gamble to escape boredom versus gambling to win money?, or 2) Do you like to gamble alone or with friends? Treatment professionals would therefore give patients two diagnoses: one based on the DSM-IV, and the other based on etiology.

2. *While the DSM is a categorical nomenclature, our new, secondary diagnosis would be indexical.* The indexical approach would work better for a diagnosis of etiology because it would provide the level of variability necessary to identify the various sub-populations of pathological gamblers, as well as find ways in which different groups are similar. More importantly, it would allow us to identify individual differences in gamblers. Having the ability to talk about pathological gambling in the aggregate, while making distinctions at the level of individual gamblers, would give the field of treatment insights heretofore unthinkable. We could explain to insurance companies and patients how they are similar to the population of pathological gamblers at large, while identifying exactly what makes each individual gambler unique. For more information on this issue see a) John Mirowsky's (1994) article "The Advantages of Indexes over Diagnoses in Scientific Assessment" in Avison and Gotlib's *Stress and Mental Health: Contemporary Issues and Prospects for the Future,* b) Mirowsky and Ross's (1989) *Social Causes of Psychological Distress,* and c) Stuart Kirk and Herb Kutchins's (1992) *The Selling of DSM: The Rhetoric of Science in Psychiatry.*

Field of Gambling Studies

1. *All of the disciplines within the social sciences, from anthropology to economics, need to get involved in the issue of pathological gambling.* A concerted effort needs to be made to get more social scientists involved in the study of pathological gambling. If we are to adopt a bio-psycho-social model, then more sociological, political and economic studies need to be done, while integrating these findings into current medical and psychological knowledge. To accomplish this agenda, people need to make a concerted effort to engage in inter-disciplinary work. Sociologists, psychologists and psychiatrists often ignore each other's work. One way to overcome this is to hold inter-disciplinary seminars and workshops where people brainstorm not on the limitations of one another's work, but on the ways in which they inform one another. The way to do this is to put

the emphasis of research on practice. Doing so makes us think of the benefits that come from different perspectives, rather than the costs. If, for example, sociologists or feminists challenge the medical model, then they should have to sit down with the medical experts they oppose to determine how best to integrate their differences into a more useful treatment approach. This is the only real way to do inter-disciplinary work. Everything else is just lip service that allows people to continue to ignore one another.

2. *More research needs to be done on pathological gambling for females, minorities, and adolescents.* In addition to doing inter-disciplinary research, we also need to place greater emphasis on how pathological gambling is a function of differences in race, class, gender, culture and age. For example, do different cultures approach the activity of gambling differently, as in the case of gambling's relevance to Asian-Americans versus Mexican-Americans versus Anglo-Americans? And, what about gambling on the Indian reservations? What impact does legalized gambling have on these people? The more sophisticated we are about these problems, the better able we are to treat this problem. For more information on gambling on Indian reservations, see Rick Hornung's (1991) *One Nation Under the Gun.* New York, Pantheon Books.

Government

Federal Government needs to address the problems of pathological gambling. Our United States government can no longer remain systematically silent about pathological gambling. It is imperative that the current National Gambling Impact Study (NGIS) make a difference. Once the NGIS is released, we should take the NGIS report and, working under the umbrella of the National Council on Problem Gambling (NCPG), construct our own formal statement specific to the problems of pathological gambling. In this way, we can hold the government accountable while setting our own agenda. For this secondary report, I make the following six recommendations:

First, *a bi-partisan formal statement needs to be written.* To construct a formal statement, the committee should include members from the National Council on Problem Gambling, state gambling council officials, recognized experts in treatment and research, members of the gambling recovery community (both families and pathological gamblers), and the gambling industry. This formal statement should be offered to the government as part of its own formal statement on drugs, alcohol, and tobacco.

Second, *this statement should start with the premise that gambling should remain legal.* The committee shouldn't get wrapped up in the problems of legalization. Make that an agenda for another committee. This committee should have as its focus the problems of pathological gambling. It should therefore start with the premise that gambling remain legal. Besides, we do not need another useless prohibition where the masses are denied their rights and freedoms.

Third, *part of our challenge should be to make government regulate the gambling industry.* We cannot continue to have government and business working hand-in-hand. Government needs to re-establish its role as government and initiate regulations that will protect the public. For more information on this issue, see Robert Goodman and Valerie Lorenz's 1994 testimonies before the House of Representatives (Goodman, Robert. 1995. "The National Impact of Casino Gambling Proliferation." *Hearing before the Committee on Small Business, House of Representatives, 103rd Congress, 2nd Session.* Washington D.C., September 21, 1994) and the NGIS web page for testimony on the issue of pathological gambling (22 January 1998, *www.ngisc.gov*).

Fourth, *government needs to fund the study, treatment, and education of pathological gambling.* Rather than coming up with new funding, government needs to make pathological gambling part of the funding it already puts aside annually to address the problems of drug addiction and alcoholism in this country. One grant through NIH is not enough. By connecting pathological gambling to these already existing funding structures, this social problem can receive the overdue funding it deserves.

Fifth, *as part of this funding structure, an investigation committee should be put together to further study the impact of pathological gambling.* This committee should again include the list of experts I stated above, along with members of the recovering community. We have available to us the efforts of state councils across the country. A grant should be given to integrate the efforts of these state councils to conduct a nation-wide study on the epidemiology of pathological gambling and its related problems.

Lastly, *the federal government needs to require that state level governments also provide support for the problems of pathological gambling.*

Like the federal government, states need to do the following: 1) put together a formal statement, 2) construct committees that include the help of councils and treatment and research experts, 3) fund studies, 4) support treatment, and 5) educate their citizens to the important problems of pathological gambling.

Gambling Industry

The Gambling Industry needs to take further responsibility for its involvement in pathological gambling. There are several important ways for the gambling industry to take responsibility for its part in the problems of pathological gambling. First, it needs to increase its financial support of state councils, research, educational programs, and treatment—for example, 1 percent of its gross profits. Second, it needs to regulate the provision of credit to people who potentially fit the pathological gambler profile. And third, it needs to educate its own staff and workers to the problems of pathological gambling so that it can protect itself as well as pathological gamblers and their families against unnecessary legal and financial problems.

The best way for the gambling industry to accomplish these tasks is to involve the assistance of experts in the fields of treatment and research, along with their local state gambling councils, people in recovery, and urban planning specialists, such as John Goodman.

Inveterate Gamblers

Our campaign to deal with the problems of pathological gambling should not infringe upon the rights of inveterate gamblers. It is important that we do not assume that everyone who gambles heavily is a pathological gambler. The majority of the population can gamble with little to no problems. Some people may gamble heavily all their lives and experience only a few temporary setbacks. When educating the general population, then, treatment professionals and researchers need to be careful of fostering a "zero-tolerance" mentality—as in the case of the war on drugs. Zero tolerance has gotten us nowhere. Let's not repeat the same mistakes when it comes to gambling.

Pathological Gamblers

1. *Pathological gamblers need to adopt a bio-psycho-social approach to their problems.* Adopting a bio-psycho-social framework is the best way for pathological gamblers to 1) become more sophisticated about their problems, 2) defend themselves in a court of law or in treatment, 3) minimize the harm they do to their families and friends, and 4) obtain the maximum amount of rights while exercising the greatest amount of responsibility. One way to accomplish this agenda is for GA and recovering people to attend conferences, ask questions, and then spread the message to others. Treatment and research experts can obviously help in this process by striving for the same agenda.

2. *Pathological gamblers need to become more active in giving voice to their problems.* Recovering pathological gamblers should involve themselves in politics so they can educate their local and federal politicians about the problems of gambling. Write to your senators, your governors, your mayors, and your city councils. They are the people voted in to protect your rights. If they won't respond to the issue, then put together petitions that challenge them to deal with the issue or face not being voted for in the next election. It is that simple. Individuals and small groups of people do have the power to make a difference.

Family

1. *Families need to adopt a bio-psycho-social approach to their problems.* Like the pathological gamblers in their lives, families need to adopt a bio-psycho-social approach to their problems. Doing so will help them in the following important ways: 1) they will finally have a discourse sophisticated enough to deal with the complexity of their problems, 2) they will have a discourse that will well represent and defend them in a court of law or in treatment, 3) it will provide them the maximum amount of rights without overemphasizing their responsibility.

Like the pathological gambler, one way to accomplish this agenda is for families to attend conferences, form your own GamAnon groups, schedule meetings with local treatment experts, ask questions, and then spread the message to others. Treatment and research experts can obviously help in this process by striving for the same agenda.

2. *Families need to become more active in giving voice to their problems.* Just like the recovering gambler (see above), families need to involve themselves in politics so they can educate their local and federal politicians about the problems of gambling. Write to your senators, your governors, your mayors, and your city councils. They are the people voted in to protect your rights.

3. *The National and State Councils should initiate a program just for the family.* Families should get involved with the national councils and their states to put together programs just for the families of pathological gamblers. Some state councils and treatment facilities are already doing this type of work. Contact the National Council for Problem Gambling to get update information on this issue (1-800-522-4700, or *www.ncpgambling.org*).

Criminal Justice System

The criminal justice system needs to adopt a bio-psycho-social approach to pathological gambling. Doing so will help them in a number of important ways.

First, *it will help them more clearly define issues of right and responsibility, and punishment and rehabilitation.* Currently, the decisions being made in courtrooms across the country are based on the strengths and weaknesses of the medical model in opposition to current law. This has got to change. The medical model isn't sophisticated enough to educate either judge or jury to the important larger and smaller situations within which any one person's gambling behavior takes place. As a result, judges and juries are making important, life-impacting decisions—and setting precedent—based only on part of the evidence.

Second, *it will help them better understand and address the problems of the family.* In all their arguments about responsibility and rights surrounding pathological gambling, lawyers have given little to no attention to the family. One way to correct this situation is to adopt a bio-psycho-social approach to the problem. In doing so, the problems of the family become immediately relevant—such as: What happens to the family if we put their loved one in jail? Are they responsible for paying the person's gambling debt? Will they make it financially? Do they have a right to sue their loved one for damages, alimony, child support?

Lastly, *adopting a bio-psycho-social approach increases the court's sophistication about the role government and the gambling industry play in the problems of pathological gambling.* If "justice" is the objective of our federal and state-level courts, then they can no longer ignore the role government and the gambling industry play in the problems of pathological gambling—as in the cases of collecting gambling-related debt or bankruptcy. Adopting a bio-psycho-social approach is one way to increase the court's sophistication about this issue because it deals with the larger social picture, while maintaining its focus on the individual.

Conclusion

As we approach the turn of the century, national awareness of pathological gambling, and the larger terms and conditions in which it is situated, is about to burst wide open. You can feel it. Change is in the air. So many smaller discursive negotiations have been taking place over the past several years which are starting to come together to form a new discursive web of awareness. The 1999 report by the NGIS Commission will set the precedent. The social sciences will become aware of the issue, funding will be made available, and pathological gambling will become an issue in congressional and state government races throughout the country. NIH and other funding agencies, like the National Center for Responsible Gaming (NCRG), are already setting the tone for the type of research and treatment that will be funded: it is still primarily medical. (In fact, all of the recent 1998 grants offered through NCRG were biomedical in focus.) We, who have been in the field now for several years, if not decades, need to think about the tone and pace we set for these larger discursive negotiations. We cannot allow these changes to be taken out of our hands and made into yet another useless "war on drugs." We have the opportunity to save billions of tax dollars and wasted efforts by demanding that pathological gambling be situated within the appropriate social, political, economic, and cultural terms and conditions in which it takes place. Action that pushes all of us toward the complexity of the issue, and not simplistic reduction, must be taken. The lives of those we care for—from pathological gamblers and their families to the communities in which we live—are at stake.

NOTES

INTRODUCTION

1. Abbott, Douglas, Sheran Cramer, and Steven Sherrets 1995. "Pathological Gambling and the Family: Practice Implications." *Families in Society,* 76(4):213–217.

2. Goodman, Robert 1995. "The National Impact of Casino Gambling Proliferation." Hearing before the Committee on Small Business, House of Representatives, 103rd Congress, 2nd Session. Washington D.C., September 21, 1994.

3. Compulsive/Problem Gamblers: Trends, Profiles, and their Importance to the Gambling Industry, located at: *web.iquest.net/cpage/ncalg/problem.htm*

4. Lorenz, Valerie 1995. "The National Impact of Casino Gambling Proliferation." Hearing before the Committee on Small Business, House of Representatives, 103rd Congress, 2nd Session. Washington D.C., September 21, 1994.

5. Goodman, Robert 1995. "The National Impact of Casino Gambling Proliferation." Hearing before the Committee on Small Business, House of Representatives, 103rd Congress, 2nd Session. Washington D.C., September 21, 1994.

6. "Beyond the Odds" in *Gambling Problems Resource Center,* page one. Located at: *www.miph.org/btosum96/whocomes.html*

7. Ibid, p. 2.

8. "Beyond the Odds" in *Gambling Problems Resource Center* page one, section two: "What happens to Families" Located at: *www.miph.org/btosum96/whathappens.html*

9. Hirshey, Gerri 1994. "Gambling Nation." *New York Times Magazine,* July 17th, p. 36.

10. Minnesota Taxes file. Located at: *www.tc.umn.edu/nlhome/g135/grosc003*

A NOTE ON STRATEGY

1. For more information, see Deleuze, Gilles 1983. *Nietzsche and Philosophy.* Page 24. New York: Columbia University Press. It is a highly regarded interpretation of Nietzsche's project. The book is also short and to the point, which makes for easy reading.

2. For more information, see Magliola, Robert 1984. *Derrida on the Mend.* Page X. Indiana: Purdue University Press. Magliola takes the work of Derrida and integrates it into certain traditions within Eastern thought, particularly Zen Buddhism.

3. For more information see Castellani, Brian 1998 "Michel Foucault and Symbolic Interactionism: The Making of a New Theory of Interaction" *Studies in Symbolic Interaction* 22, 247–272. In this article I explain the differences between a Foucaultian and symbolic interactionist conception of domination and how I differ from these perspectives through my usage of Strauss' concept of negotiation and negotiated order.

4. For more information on Strauss' concept of negotiation, see Strauss, Anselm 1978. *Negotiations: Varieties, Contexts, Processes, and Social Order.* Page IX. San Francisco: Jossey-Bass Publishers.

CHAPTER ONE

1. For more information, see United States Court of Appeals for the Second Circuit, docket No. 83–1459, "United States of America v. John J. Torniero," Appellee's Brief p. 3.

2. For more information, see United States Court of Appeals for the Second Circuit, docket No. 83–1459, "United States of America v. John J. Torniero," Appellee's Brief p. 3.

3. At the time of Bergler's texts, there were other articles being published as well. Most of them were in reaction to or built off of Bergler's work. One of the

more important was Greenson's 1947 article "On Gambling" in the *American Imago*. The American editor was Dr. Hanns Sachs of Boston, Massachusetts. Of course there is Freud's famous analysis of Dostoevsky "Dostoevski and Patricide" (*Gesammelte Schriften*, XII: 8–26, 1928). Other articles included Robert Linder's "The Psychodynamics of Gambling," found in *The Annals of the American Academy of Political And Social Science,* May 1950, and Iago Galdston's "The Psychodynamics of the Triad—Alcoholism, Gambling and Superstition" (lecture delivered at the New York Academy of Medicine, March, 1951). See also Bergler (1958, pp 80–81) for more information. All of these articles, in one way or another, acted as historical markers for the expansion of the medical model to include pathological gambling.

4. For more information, see Findlay's (1986) *"People of Chance"* and Rose's (1986) book "*Gambling and the Law*" Chapter I ("The Spread of Legalized Gambling"). Gambling was legal during the establishment of the thirteen Colonies in the United States. It was then made illegal in the early 1800s throughout most of the country, with the exception of the Western frontier. The second wave of legalized gambling started shortly before the Civil War as a way to amend various failing state economies. Because of massive corruption, shortly after the Civil War, all of the states once again decided to make it illegal for the second time—except in Louisiana. Louisiana had one of the most corrupt state gambling organizations in the country and had no interest in shutting itself down. In 1890, because of the Louisiana Lottery Scandal, the federal government stepped in and made all forms of gambling illegal. The laws for the late 1800s remained in tact until 1963. The only exceptions to this were Las Vegas, which built its first casinos in the 1930s, and New Jersey.

5. For more information on the debate, see *The Herald* web site *www.sharonherald. com/govt/eln1196/ gambb103096.html.* The article titles are a) *Youngstown Would Get 1 of 8 Riverboat Casinos* and b) *Gambling Casinos may Encircle Pennsylvania.* Both articles are by Robert Swift.

CHAPTER TWO

1. To read more about the controversial rulings regarding addiction and the insanity defense see a) Insanity Defense Work Group. 1983. "American Psychiatric Association Statement on the Insanity Defense." *American Journal of Psychiatry,* 140(6):681–688 and b) Paul S. Appelbaum. 1994. *Almost a Revolution: Mental Health Law and the Limits of Change.* New York: Oxford University Press.

CHAPTER FOUR

1. United States of America v. John Torniero, No. 83–1459, Brief for the Appellant, p. 15. United States Court of Appeals for the Second Circuit.

2. Ibid, p. 16.

3. Ibid, p. 17.

4. Ibid, p. 16.

5. Ibid, pp. 18–19.

6. Ibid, p. 18.

7. Ibid, p. 19.

8. Ibid, p. 19.

9. Ibid, p. 19.

10. Ibid, p. 19.

11. Ibid, p. 17.

12. Ibid, p. 20.

13. Ibid, p. 20.

14. Ibid, p. 16.

15. Ibid, p. 22.

16. Ibid, p. 22.

17. Ibid, p. 23.

18. Ibid, p. 23.

19. Ibid, p. 23.

20. Ibid, p. 23.

21. Ibid, p. 23–24.

22. Ibid, p. 25.

23. Ibid, pp. 25–26.

24. Ibid, p. 26.

25. Ibid, p. 38.

CHAPTER SIX

1. For information on the various state councils, see the National Council's web page at *www.ncpgambling.org*, or call the National Council at 1–800–330–8739.

2. Again, because of problems of negotiation and because of potential conflicts and differences of opinion, some of the more hard-core GA members are against the control of the medical institute. They see its involvement with GA as potentially damaging. Along with the more hard-core members of GA, there are treatment experts who don't think GA really works, nor do they think that much if any psychological or psychiatric treatment works either. For example, Taber, the author of this survey, wrote an article, "Common Characteristics of Pathological Gamblers and Some Interventions which Seem to Help" (1983). This article is a polemic against the idea that medical treatment can actually categorize, find similarities across gamblers, diagnose, and cure the excesses and problems of gambling. He argues instead that the most we can hope for are some similar characteristics between pathological gamblers that allow us to help them. But, each person should be approached on a case by case basis. It is also important to note that Taber did, for a while, during the late 1970s and early 1980s run the Gambling Treatment Program at the Brecksville VA Medical Center. However, as this survey shows, and as I explained in chapter two regarding the dimensional model, Taber's philosophy of gambling is not widely shared, and is, for the most part—both within the field of gambling studies and GA—in the strong minority.

CHAPTER SEVEN

1. United States vs. John J. Torniero, 1983 Criminal 82–1106, pp. 94–97.

2. United States of America v. John Torniero, No. 83–1459, Brief for the Appellee, p. 7. United States Court of Appeals for the Second Circuit.

3. Ibid, p. 11.

CHAPTER NINE

1. This chapter should be read in conjunction with two chapters from Goodman's (1995) *The Luck Business*. These are chapter five, "Chaser Governments: The Accidental Gambling Entrepreneurs," and chapter eight, "The Government as Predator: A Troubling New Role in Troubled Economies."

2. See the Boshard's 6 June 97 article in the *Gazette, www.gazetteonline.com.*

3. For more information about statistics see Goodman (1995) and go through the latest editions of *Gaming and Wagering Business,* which is always providing updated statistics.

4. For information on annual expenditures see the *National Review* essays by William F. Buckley and others at *www.xs4all.nl/~mlap/special/wodbuc.html.*

5. For more information on incarceration rates and the relationship between drugs and crime see Drugs and Crime: Evaluating Public Policy Initiatives, edited by Doris Layton MacKenzie and Craig Uchida (1994), Poor Discipline: Parole and the Social Control of the Underclass, 1890–1990, by Jonathan Simon (1993), The Politics of Alcoholism, by Carolyn Wiener (1981), and the *National Review* essays by William F. Buckley and others at *www.xs4all.nl/~mlap/special/wodbuc.html.*

6. For more information on Clinton's drug plan see CNN—"Clinton Presents Five-Step Drug Plan," 29 April 1996, *www.cnn.com/US/9604/29/clinton.miami/clinton.drug.2/index.html.* For information on the Bush and Reagan plan see *turnpike.net/-jnr/bushwar.htm.*

7. From phone interview with attorney, Paul Ash, President of the National Council on Problem Gambling.

8. These outcome results come from a study done by the state of Minnesota on six state-supported compulsive gambling treatment programs. For an in-depth review of the statistics, see the study's web site at: *www.cbc.med.umn.edu/~randy/gambling/gamtx.htm.*

REFERENCES

A., Paul, Esq. 1988. "Recovery, Reinstatement, Serenity: The Personal Account Of A Compulsive Gambler." *Journal of Gambling Behavior,* 4(4):312–315.

American Psychiatric Association 1980. *Diagnostic Statistical Manual of Mental Disorders, (Third Edition).* Washington, DC: American Psychiatric Association

American Psychiatric Association 1987. *Diagnostic Statistical Manual of Mental Disorders, (Third Edition, Revised).* Washington, DC: American Psychiatric Association

American Psychiatric Association 1994. *Diagnostic Statistical Manual of Mental Disorders, Fourth Edition.* Washington, DC: American Psychiatric Association

Barton, Babette B. 1990. "Legal And Tax Incidents Of Compulsive Behavior: Lessons From Zarin." *The Tax Lawyer,* 45:749–782.

Bergler, Edmund 1943. "The Gambler: A Misunderstood Neurotic." *Criminal Psychopathology,* 4(3): 379–393.

Bergler, Edmund 1958. *The Psychology Of Gambling.* London: Bernard Hanison Limited.

Berman, Linda and Mary-Ellen Siegel 1992. *Behind The 8-Ball: A Guide For Families Of Gamblers.* New York: A Fireside/Parkside Recovery Book, Published by Simon and Schuster

Black, Donald, Rise Goldstein, Russell Noyes, and Nancee Blum 1994. "Compulsive Behaviors And Obsessive-Compulsive Disorder (OCD): Lack Of A Relationship Between OCD, Eating Disorders, And Gambling." *Comprehensive Psychiatry,* 35(2):145–148.

Blanco, Carlos, Luis Orensanz-Munoz, Carmen Blanco-Jerez, and Jeronimo Saiz-Ruiz 1996. "Pathological Gambling And Platelet MAO Activity: A Psychobiological Study." *American Journal of Psychiatry,* 153(1):119–121.

Blaszczynski, Alex 1985. "Pathological Gambling: An Illness Or Myth." In J.

McMillen (Ed.), *Gambling In The 80s.* Proceedings of the inaugural conference of the National Association for Gambling Studies (NAGS), Brisbane.

Blaszczynski, Alex and Neil McConaghy 1989. "The Medical Model Of Pathological Gambling: Current Shortcomings." *Journal of Gambling Behavior,* 5(1):42–52.

Blaszczynski, Alex and Neil McConaghy 1994. "Criminal Offenses in Gamblers Anonymous and Hospital Treated Pathological Gamblers." *Journal of Gambling Studies,* 10(2): 99–127.

Blaszczynski, A., N. McConaghy and A. Frankova 1989. "Crime, Antisocial Personality and Pathological Gambling." *Journal of Gambling Behavior,* 5(2):137–152.

Blaszczynski, A., N. McConaghy and A. Frankova 1991. "Control Versus Abstinence In The Treatment Of Pathological Gambling: A Two To Nine Year Follow-up." *British Journal of Addiction,* 86: 299–306.

Blaszczynski, Alex P., Neil McConaghy, and S. Winter 1986. "Plasma Endorphin Levels In Pathological Gambling." *Journal of Gambling Behavior,* 2:3–14.

Blaszczynski, Alex and Derrick Silove 1995. "Cognitive And Behavioral Therapies For Pathological Gambling." *Journal of Gambling Studies,* 11(2):195–220.

Blume, Sheila 1987. "Compulsive Gambling And The Medical Model." *The Journal of Gambling Behavior,* 3(4): 237–247.

Bradshaw, Jon 1975. *Fast Company.* NY: Harper's Magazine Press.

Bybee, Shannon 1988. "Problem Gambling: One View From The Gambling Industry Side." *Journal of Gambling Behavior,* 4(4):301–308.

Carlton, Peter and Leonide Goldstein 1987. "Physiological Determinants Of Pathological Gambling." In Thomas Galski's (Ed.) *The Handbook of Pathological Gambling.* Springfield IL: Charles C. Thomas.

Carlton, Peter and Paul Manowitz 1992. "Behavioral Restraint And Symptoms Of Attention Deficit Disorder In Alcoholics And Pathological Gamblers." *Neuropsychobiology,* 25(1):44–48.

Carlton, Peter, Paul Manowitz, Herbert McBride, and Rena Nora 1987. "Attention Deficit Disorder And Pathological Gambling." *Journal of Clinical Psychiatry,* 48(12):487–488.

Carrasco, Jose Luis, J. Saiz-Ruiz, Eric Hollander, J. Cesar 1994. "Low Platelet Monoamine Oxidase Activity In Pathological Gambling." *Acta Psychiatrica Scandinavica,* 90(6): 427–431.

Carroll, Douglas and Justine Huxley 1994. "Cognitive, Dispositional, And Psychobiological Correlates Of Dependent Slot Machine Gambling In Young People." *Journal of Applied Social Psychology,* 24(12):1070–1083.

Castellani, Brian 1999. "Foucault and Symbolic Interactionism: The Making of a New Theory of Interaction." *Studies in Symbolic Interaction,* 22, 247–272.

Castellani, Brian and Lori Rugle 1995. "A Comparison Of Pathological Gamblers To Alcoholics And Cocaine Misusers On Impulsivity, Sensation Seeking, And Craving." *The International Journal of the Addictions* 30:275–289.

Cloulombe, Andress, Robert Ladouceur, Raymond Desharnais, and Jean Jobin 1992. "Erroneous Perceptions And Arousal Among Regular And Occasional Video Poker Players." *Journal of Gambling Studies,* 8(3):235–244.

Cocco, Nick, Louise Sharpe, and Alex Blaszczynski 1995. "Differences In Preferred Level Of Arousal In Two Sub-Groups Of Problem Gamblers: A Preliminary Report." *Journal of Gambling Studies,* 11(2):221–229.

Comings, David, Richard Rosenthal, Henry Lesieur, Loreen Rugle, Donn Muhleman, Connie Chiu, George Dietz, and Radhika Gade 1996. "A Study of the Dopamine D2 Receptor Gene in Pathological Gambling." *Pharmacogenetics,* 6:223–234.

Comings, David, R. Gade, S. Wu, C. Chiu, G. Dietz, D. Muhleman, G. Saucier, L. Ferry, R. Rosenthal, H. Lesieur, L. Rugle, and P. MacMurray 1997. "Studies of the Potential Role of the Dopamine D1 Receptor Gene in Addictive Behaviors." *Molecular Psychiatry,* 2(1):44–56.

Conrad P. and W. Schneider 1980. *Deviance And Medicalization: From Badness To Sickness.* St. Louis MO: Mosby.

Cunnien, Alan J. 1985. "Pathological Gambling As An Insanity Defense." *Behavioral Sciences and the Law,* 3 (Winter):85–101.

Custer, R. L. and H. Milt 1985. *When Luck Runs Out.* New York: Facts on File Publications.

Dickerson, Mark 1979. "FI Schedules And Persistence At Gambling In The UK Betting Office." *Journal of Applied Behavioral Analysis,* 12:315–323.

Dickerson, Mark 1984. *Compulsive Gamblers.* London: Longman.

Dickerson, Mark 1993. Internal And External Determinants Of Persistence Gambling: Problems In Generalizing From One Form Of Gambling To Another." *Journal of Gambling Studies,* 9(3):225–245.

Dickerson M., and D. Weeks 1979. "Controlled Gambling As A Therapeutic Technique For Compulsive Gamblers." *Journal of Behavior Therapy and Experimental Psychiatry,* 10:139–141.

Douglas and Huxley 1994. "Cognitive, Dispositional, and Psychobiological Correlates of Dependent Slot Machine Gambling in Young People." *Journal of Applied Social Psychology,* 24(2): 1070–1083.

Foucault, Michel 1965. *Madness And Civilization: A History Of Insanity In The Age Of Reason.* New York: Vintage Books.

Foucault, Michel 1972. *The Archeology Of Knowledge.* New York: Harper.

Foucault, Michel 1979. *Discipline And Punish: The Birth Of The Prison.* New York: Vintage Books.

Foucault, Michel 1988. *Technologies Of The Self: A Seminar With Michel Foucault.* Edited by Luther Martin, Huck Gutman, and Patrick Hutton. Amherst: University of Massachusetts Press.

Gamblers Anonymous 1989. *Gamblers Anonymous: A New Beginning.* Los Angeles: Gamblers Anonymous.

Gamblers Anonymous 1984. *Sharing Recovery Through Gamblers Anonymous.* Los Angeles: Gamblers Anonymous Publishing Inc.

Gerhardt, Utah 1989. *Ideas About Illness: An Intellectual And Political History Of Medical Sociology.* New York: New York University Press.

Gifis, Steven 1991. *Law Dictionary, Third Edition.* New York: Barrons.

Glaser, B. and A. Strauss 1968. *The Discovery of Grounded Theory, Strategies for Qualitative Research.* London: Weidenfeld and Nicolson.

Gleick, James 1987. *Chaos: The Making of a New Science.* New York: Penguin Books.

Goffman, Erving 1963. *Stigma: Note on the Management of Spoiled Identity.* Garden City, New York: Simon & Schuster.

Goldstein, Leonide and Peter Carlton 1988. "Hemispheric EEG Correlates Of Compulsive Behavior: The Case Of Pathological Gamblers." *Research Communications in Psychology, Psychiatry & Behavior,* 13(1–2):103–111.

Goodman, Robert 1995. *The Luck Business: The Devastating Consequences And Broken Promises Of America's Gambling Explosion.* New York: Free Press Paperbacks.

Griffiths, Mark 1989. "Psychobiology Of The Near-Miss In Fruit Machine Gambling." *Journal of Psychology,* 125(3):347–357.

Griffiths, Mark 1995. *Adolescent Gambling.* New York: Routledge.

Haller, Reinhard and H. Hinterhuber 1994. "Treatment Of Pathological Gambling With Carbamazepine." *Pharmacopsychiatry,* 27(3):129.

Halpern, Abraham 1977. "The Insanity Defense: A Judicial Anachronism"

Halpern, Abraham 1980. "The Fiction of Legal Insanity and the Misuse of Psychiatry."

Heineman, Mary 1992. *Losing Your Shirt: Recovery For Compulsive Gamblers And Their Families.* Minneapolis: CompCare Publishers.

Hirshey, Gerri 1994. "Gambling Nation." *New York Times Magazine,* July 17th, p. 36.

Hollander, Eric, Maxim Frenkel, Concetta Decaria, Sari Trungold, et al. 1992. "Treatment Of Pathological Gambling With Clomipramine." *American Journal of Psychiatry,* 149(5):710–711.

Insanity Defense Work Group 1983. "American Psychiatric Association Statement on the Insanity Defense." *American Journal of Psychiatry,* 140(6):681–688.

Jarvis, Stephan 1988. "From the View of a Compulsive Gambler/Recidivist." *Journal of Gambling Behavior,* 4(4):316–319.

Kaplan, Harold, Benjamin Sadock and Jack Grebb 1994. *Kaplan and Sadock's Synopsis of Psychiatry: Behavioral Sciences, Clinical Psychiatry (7th ed.)*. Baltimore, MD: Williams & Wilkins Co.

Kennedy, David. 1994. "Gambling And The Bankruptcy Discharge: An Historical Exegesis And Case Survey." *Bankruptcy Developments Journal,* 11:49–84.

Kroeber, Hans-Ludwig 1992. "Roulette Gamblers And Gamblers At Electronic Game Machines: Where Are The Differences?" *Journal of Gambling Studies,* 8(1):79–92.

Lesieur, Henry 1977. *The Chase: Career of a Compulsive Gambler.* New York: Anchor Books

Lesieur, Henry and Richard Rosenthal 1991. "A Review Of The Literature (Prepared For The American Psychiatric Association Task Force On DSM-IV Committee On Disorders Of Impulse Control Not Elsewhere Classified." *Journal of Gambling Studies,* 7 (1): 5–39.

Lesieur, Henry and Sheila Blume 1987. "The South Oaks Gambling Screen (SOGS): A New Instrument for The Identification Of Pathological Gamblers." *American Journal of Psychiatry,* 144(9):1184–1188.

Lesieur, Henry and Sheila Blume 1990. "Characteristics Of Pathological Gamblers Identified Among Patients On A Psychiatric Admissions Service." *Hospital and Community Psychiatry,* 41(9):1009–1012.

Lesieur, Henry and Sheila Blume 1992. "Modifying The Addiction Severity Index for use with Pathological Gamblers." *American Journal on Addictions,* 1(3):240–247.

Lewis, Albert 1986. "Collection Of Gambling Debt." *New York State Bar Journal,* 58:24–26.

Maines, D. and J. Charlton 1985. "The Negotiated Order Approach to the Analysis of Social Organization" pp. 271–308 in *Foundations of Interpretive Sociology: Original Essays in Symbolic Interactions,* edited by H. Farberman and R. Perinbauayagam. Greenwich, CT: JAI Press.

McConaghy, Nathaniel 1991. "A Pathological Or A Compulsive Gambler? *Journal of Gambling Studies,* 7(1): 55–64.

McCormick, Richard 1988. "Attributional Style In Pathological Gamblers In Treatment." *Journal of Abnormal Psychology,* 97(3):368–370.

Moreno, I, J. Saiz-Ruiz, J. Lopez-Ibor 1991. "Serotonin And Gambling Dependence." *Human Pychopharmacology,* 6:9–12.

Oldman, David 1978. "Compulsive Gamblers." *Sociological Review,* 26:349–371.

Ottinger, Paul William 1988. "The Early Warning System That Failed: A Personal Account." *Journal of Gambling Behavior,* 4(4):309–311.

P., Bernie and William Bruns 1973. *Compulsive Gambler.* Secaucus NJ: Lyle Suart, Inc

Perez de Castro, I., A. Ibanez, P. Torres, J. Saiz-Ruiz, and J. Fernandez-Piqueras

1997. "Genetic Association Study Between Pathological Gambling and a Functional DNA Polymorphism at the D4 Receptor Gene." *Pharmacogenetics,* 7(5):345–348.

Rachlin, Stephen, Abraham L. Halpern, and Stanley L. Protnow 1986. "Pathological Gambling And Criminal Responsibility." *Journal of Forensic Sciences,* 31 (January):235–240.

Ramirez, Luis, Richard McCormick, and Martin Lowy 1988. "Plasma Cortisol And Depression In Pathological Gamblers." *British Journal of Psychiatry,* 153: 684–686.

Roby, Kevin 1995. "Effects of Accuracy Feedback Versus Monetary Contingency On Arousal In High And Low Frequency Gamblers." *Journal of Gambling Studies,* 11(2):185–193.

Rose, I. Nelson 1988. "Compulsive Gambling and the Law: From Sin to Vice to Disease." *Journal of Gambling Behavior,* 4(4): 240–260.

Rosecrance, John 1985a. "Compulsive Gambling and The Medicalization of Deviance." *Social Problems* 32(3):275–284.

Rosecrance, John 1985b. *The Degenerates of Lake Tahoe: A Study of Persistence in the Social World of Horse Race Gambling.* New York: Peter Laing.

Rosecrance, John 1986a. "Attributions and the Origins of Problem Gambling." *The Sociological Quarterly* 27(4):463–477.

Rosecrance, John 1986b. "Why Regular Gamblers Don't Quit: A Sociological Perspective." *Sociological Perspectives,* 29(3), 357–378.

Rosecrance, John 1988. *Gambling Without Guilt: The Legitimation of an American Pastime.* California: Brooks/Cole Publishing Company.

Rosecrance, John 1989. "Controlled Gambling: A Promising Future." In Howard J. Shaffer, Sharon A. Stein, and Blase Gambino's (Eds.) *Compulsive Gambling: Theory, Research, and Practice.* Massachusetts: Lexington Books.

Rosenthal, Richard and Valerie Lorenz 1992. "The Pathological Gambler as Criminal Offender." Clinical Forensic Psychiatry, 15(3):647–660.

Roy, Alec 1991. "Cerebrospinal Fluid Diazepam Binding Inhibitor In Depressed Patients And Normal Controls: A Novel Peptide With Multiple Functions." *Neuropharmacology,* 30(12B):1441–1444.

Roy, Alec, Bryon Adinoff, Laurie Roehrich, Danuta Lamparski et al. 1989. "Pathological Gambling: A Psychobiological Study." *Archives of General Psychiatry,* 45(4): 369–373.

Roy, Alec, Judith DeJong, Thomas Ferraro, Bryon Adinoff, et al. 1989. "CSF GABA And Neuropeptides In Pathological Gamblers And Normal Controls." *Psychiatry Research,* 30(2):137–144.

Roy, Alec, D. Picker, P. Gold, M. Barbaccia, et al. 1989. "Diazepam-binding Inhibitor And Corticotropin-Releasing Hormone In Cerebrospinal Fliud." *Acta Psychiatrica Scandinavica,* 80(3):287–291.

Roy, Alec, D., Wade Berrettine, Bryon Adinoff, and Markku Linnoila 1990. "CSF Galin In Alcoholics, Pathological Gamblers, And Normal Controls: A Negative Report." *Biological Psychiatry,* 27(8):923–926.

Rubin, Ann 1982. "Beating the Odds: Compulsive Gambling as an Insanity Defense." *Connecticut Law Review,* 14:341–367.

Rugle, Loreen 1993. Initial Thoughts on Viewing Pathological Gambling from a Physiological and Intrapsychic Structural Perspective." *Journal of Gambling Studies,* 9(1): 3–16.

Rugle, Loreen and Lawrence Melamed 1993. "Neuropsychological Assessment Of Attention Problems In Pathological Gamblers." *The Journal of Nervous And Mental Disease,* 181(2):107–112.

Sharpe, Loiuse and Tarrier Nicholas 1992. "A Cognitive-Behavioral Treatment Approach For Problem Gambling." *Journal of Cognitive Psychotherapy: International Quarterly,* 6(3):193–203.

Sharpe, Loiuse and Tarrier Nicholas 1995. "Towards A Cognitive-Behavioral Theory Of Problem Gambling." *British Journal of Psychiatry,* 162:407–412.

Sharpe, Loiuse, Nicholas Tarrier, David Schotte, and Susan Spence 1995. "The Role Of Autonomic Gambling Arousal In Problem Gambling." *Addiction,* 90(11): 1529–1540.

Specker, Sheila, Gregory Carlson, Gary Christenson and Michael Marcotte 1995. "Impulse control disorders and attention deficit disorder in pathological gamblers." *Annals of Clinical Psychiatry,* 7(4):175–179.

Strauss, Anslem 1978. *Negotiations: Varieties, Contexts, Processes, And Social Order.* San Francisco: Jossey-Bass Publishers.

Strauss, Anselm 1993. *Continual Permutations Of Action.* New York: Aldine De Gruyter.

Templer, Donald, George Kaiser and Karen Siscoe 1993. "Correlates of Pathological Gambling Propensity in Prison Inmates." *Comprehensive Psychiatry,* 34(5):347–153.

Turner, Bryan S. 1987. *Medical Power And Social Knowledge.* CA: Sage. *United States v. Lafferty,* 189 Conn. 360, 456A.2d 272 (1983); 192 Conn 571, 472 A.2d 1275 (1984).

United States v. Lewellyn, 723 F.2d 615 (8th Cir. 1983).

United States v. Torniero, 570 F. Supp. 721 (2d Cir. 1983).

United States v. Torniero, 735 F.2d 725. (2nd Cir. 1984).

United States of America v. John Torniero, No. 83–1459, Brief for the Appellee. United States Court of Appeals for the Second Circuit 1984.

United States of America v. John Torniero, No. 83–1459, Brief for the Appellant. United States Court of Appeals for the Second Circuit 1984.

United States vs. John J. Torniero, 1983 Criminal Docket 82–1106.

Volberg, Rachel 1994. "The Prevelance and Demographics of Pathological Gamblers: Implications for Public Health." *American Journal of Public Health,* 84(2):237–241.

Volberg, Rachel and Henry Steadman 1988. "Refining Prevalence Estimates Of Pathological Gambling." *American Journal of Psychiatry,* 145(4): 502–505.

Wedgeworth, Raymond 1998. "The Reification of the 'Pathological' Gambler: An Analysis of Gambling Treatment and the Application of the Medical Model to Problem Gambling." *Perspectives in Psychiatric Care,* 34(2): 5–13.

Wolfe, Joy 1995. "Casinos And The Compulsive Gambler: Is There A Duty To Monitor The Gambler's Wagers?" *Mississippi Law Journal,* 64:687–701.

Yes on Issue 1 Committee 1996. *Ohio Issue 1 Limited Riverboat Gambling: 1996 Voter Fact Book.* Columbus, OH: Yes on Issue 1 Committee

Zola, Irving 1972. "Medicine as an Institute of Social Control: The Medicalizing of Society." *The Sociological Review,* 20(4):487–504.

Zorn, Stephen 1995. "The Federal Income Tax Treatment Of Gambling: Fairness Or Obsolete Moralism?" *The Tax Lawyer,* 49:1–54.

INDEX

Assemblage
in art, 10
definition of, 10–11
outline of method, 7–11
vertical versus lateral thinking, 8–10
See also Discursive negotiations
Attention deficit disorder and impulsivity. *See* Pathological gambling, neuropsychology of

Bergler, Edmund, 23–24, 25, 27–29, 91
Blaszczynski, Alex, 28, 49, 59, 61, 63, 173, 174, 175, 195
Blume, Sheila, 38, 61, 78, 79–81, 84, 102
Bybee, Shannon, 125–132

Comings, David, 49, 59, 64–65
Conrad, Peter, 37, 49, 50, 51, 59, 78, 80, 87, 104
Court cases
overview of cases, 22–23
United States v. Campanaro, 22
United States v. Lafferty, 22
United States v. Lewellyn, 22, 113–114
United States v. Torniero. *See under* United States v. Torniero
See also Criminal justice system; Insanity defense
Criminal justice system, 8, 23–25, 27–29, 38–40, 41–48. *See also* Court cases; Insanity defense; United States v. Torniero
improving the care of gambling related crimes, 203–204
Custer, Robert, 26–27, 67–68, 70–72, 74, 75, 78, 81–82, 86, 88, 91–98, 153

Deleuze, Gilles, 11
Derrida, Jacques, 11
Diagnostic and Statistical Manual of Mental Disorders (DSM), 52–57. *See also* Medical model of pathological gambling
improvement of, 197–198
Discursive negotiations
confession as negotiation, 150–151, 157–159
definition of, 12
discursive agency, 80–81, 86–90, 93–98
discursive strategies, 80–81, 84–86, 93–98
example of, 12–15, 87–90, 91–98

improvisational nature of negotiation, 14
interaction as negotiation, 12, 86
legal exam as negotiation, 41–46
negotiated order, 82–83, 90, 155–156
organizing practice, outlined, 90–91
outline of theory, 11–16, 80–91
power and domination as negotiation, 13–15, 83, 84, 85, 87
resistance as negotiation, 14–15, 156
social structure and its limitations, 84, 86–90
two-fold process of interaction, 81, 90, 93
See also Assemblage
Domination. *See* Discursive Negotiations, power and domination as negotiation
DSM. *See* Diagnostic and Statistical Manual of Mental Disorders
Dunne, Joseph (Monsignor), 67, 74, 75, 100

Family
children, 178, 184–185
and the criminal justice system, 181–182
and Gamblers Anonymous (GA), 184
and the gambling industry, 179–180
and the government, 178
impact of pathological gambling, 4, 71, 177–185
improving the care of, 202–203
and the medical model of pathological gambling, 183–184
spouse, first-person accounts, 3–4, 178, 179, 180–181, 182–183, 184–185
treatment, 95, 183–184
Field of gambling studies, 49, 51–52, 60–66
improvement of, 198–199
Foucault, Michel, 15, 37, 44, 149, 156–157

GA. *See* Gamblers Anonymous
Gamblers Anonymous (GA), 25–26, 77, 78, 93–94, 99–103, 194
Gambling councils, 99, 103–104. *See also* National Center for Responsible Gaming; National Council on Problem Gambling
Gambling industry, 4, 29, 36–37, 123–134, 179–181, 201
improvement of, 201
involvement in treatment, 103–104, 133–134
overview of, 123–134
percentage of population involved in gambling, 36–37
replacing pathological gambling with problem gambling, 131–132
revenue, examples of, 4, 29, 33, 36–37, 137
spread of casinos, 29
views toward pathological gambling, 123–134
Genetics. *See* Pathological gambling, genetics of
Goodman, Robert, 6, 29–30, 31–32, 37, 106, 124, 133, 137–138, 200, 201
Government
funding for treatment and research. *See* National Institutes of Health (NIH)
improvement of, 199–201
legalization of gambling, 29–35
revenue from lotteries, examples, 33, 137
taxation of gambling industry, 4
views toward gambling, 135–142

Insanity defense
American Law Institute (ALI) definition of, 46–48, 68–69, 72, 75, 119–121
and the DSM diagnosis of pathological gambling, 111–117
Insanity Defense Work Group, 47, 108, 114–115
legal versus clinical definitions of insanity, 54–55, 108–109, 117–121
See also Court cases; Criminal justice system; United States v. Torniero
Inveterate Gamblers
changing society's and treatment expert's attitude's toward, 201
overview of, 161–175
successful versus failed gambling, 168–171
views toward the medical model of pathological gambling, 168–170

Johnston, William, 11
Journal of Gambling Studies, 21, 51, 100, 126, 144

Lesieur, Henry, 55–56, 57, 79, 88, 142, 170
Lorenz, Valerie, 28, 136, 200

Magliola, Robert, 11
Medical model of pathological gambling and the criminal justice system. *See* Criminal justice system; Insanity defense
definition of, 50–52, 79–80
and the DSM, 52–57, 58, 65–66, 80, 86, 197–198
and Gamblers Anonymous (GA), 101–103
historical context of, 20–22, 23–27, 37–38
improvement of, 193–194
usage in research, 51–52, 57–66
usage in treatment, 77–79, 91–98
See also Pathological gambling
Method of book. *See* Assemblage

National Center for Responsible Gaming, 140, 204
National Council on Problem Gambling, 67, 100, 103–104, 194, 199, 203
National Gambling Impact Study, 141–142, 199, 200, 204
National Institute on Drug Abuse (NIDA), 5, 139, 140
National Institutes of Health (NIH), 139, 140, 200, 204
NIDA. *See* National Institute on Drug Abuse
Nietzsche, Friedrich, 11
NIH. *See* National Institutes of Health

Oldman, David, 171–172, 174

Pathological Gamblers
and the act of medical confession to others, 148–157
and the act of medical confession to self, 157–159
first-person accounts, 144–148, 161–167
improving the care of, 202
views toward the criminal justice system, 151–159
See also Pathological gambling
Pathological Gambling
comorbidity, 71, 140–141
compliance with treatment, 155
criminal behavior, 4, 73–75, 110–111. *See also* Insanity defense
Diagnostic and Statistical Manual of Mental Disorders (DSM) diagnosis of, 20–21, 35, 38–39, 52–58, 73, 108, 110–115, 187. *See also* Medical model of pathological gambling

financial debt, 4
gender differences, 3, 178
genetics of, 49, 64–65, 194
middle-class, 36–37
neuropsychology of, 61–62
percentage of adolescents, 3, 37, 196
percentage of United States adult population, 3, 36–37
psychophysiology of, 62–63
severity of, 69–72, 111
social costs, 3–4, 35–36
See also Medical model of pathological gambling
Postmodernism. *See* Discursive negotiations
Poststructuralism. *See* Foucault, Michel; Discursive negotiations
Power/Knowledge (Foucault). *See* Discursive negotiations

Research, pathological gambling. *See* Field of gambling studies
Resistance. *See* Discursive negotiations, resistance as negotiation
Revenue, from gambling. *See* Gambling industry; Government
Rose, I. Nelson, 21–22, 23, 39, 104, 118, 125, 126, 144, 180, 181, 187–188
Rosecrance, John, 26, 36, 57, 100, 103, 168, 170–172, 174–175
Rosenthal, Richard, 28, 55–56, 88
Rugle, Loreen, 49, 59, 61, 88

Schneider, Joseph. *See* Conrad, Peter
Shaffer, Howard, 124, 141–142
Sociology of knowledge. *See* Conrad, Peter; Discursive negotiations; Foucault, Michel
Strauss, Anselm, 15, 155
Symbolic interactionism. *See* Discursive negotiations; Strauss, Anselm

Taber, Julian, 70, 71, 72, 74, 75, 101–103
Theory of book. *See* Discursive negotiations
Treatment
Brecksville Gambling Treatment Program, 5, 6, 26–27, 68, 91–98, 129, 130
brief history of, 26–27
Custer's in-patient medical model approach, 91–98
dimensional (cognitive-behavioral) model of pathological gambling, 172–174
and the family. *See* Family
improvement of, 194–197
Rosecrance's controlled gambling approach, 171–172
See also Medical model of pathological gambling

United States v. Torniero
defense's argument, 67–75
judge's decision, 187–190
nature of the crime, 19–20
prosecution's argument, 107–121
review of the pre-trial hearing, 41–48
See also Court cases; Criminal justice system

Volberg, Rachel, 36

Wedgeworth, Raymond, 105, 170, 184